# CHILD HEALTH NURSING

# CHILD HEALTH NURSING

Sanjeev Singh

genNEXT Publication

Child Health Nursing

Rs. 890



ISBN: 978-81-908675-0-4.



Published in 2010 in India by
Gennext Publication
23 Main Ansari Road, Darya Ganj,
New Delhi-110002
E-Mail:GenNextpublication@hotmail.com
Phone: 23282060

*Printed at:* Singhal Print Media, Delhi

# Contents

# Preface

Nurses play a key role in the health care delivery system. Nursing is considered to be an important profession for which a strong preparation is needed. This textbook is written for the nurse students who have to learn and excel in the field of child health. This book is framed considering the syllabus given and revised by the Nursing Council of India and the additional requirement for education and training.

This book is written and reviewed by the experts in the field of nursing and also by teachers teaching in the renowned nursing colleges and institutes. Much emphasis is given to practical approaches as the students are expected to demonstrate skill in their practice in actual situations.

The child health nursing is an expanding area as a result of the broadening scope of practice within the nursing profession and the recognized need for better preventive and restorative care in these areas. The importance of this need is reûected in the fact that many of the year 2010 health goals for the nation focus on these areas of nursing.

At the same time that the information in these areas of nursing is increasing, less time is available in nursing programs to cover it. Students experience difûculty reading all of the material available in the market. So I here put my efforts and experience to capsule the whole syllabus of Nursing in this book including all the topics in a precise but comprehensible manner. Undersigned is confident enough that this book will be a handy tool in the students of nursing. Your sincere feedback always encourage me to improve my way of presentation. Reader's suggestions and comments are always welcome.

# 1

# Introduction

Child health nursing is a field of nursing and medical practice with a focus on rendering complete care to infants, children and adolescents. It is different from paediatrics, therein the stress in paediatrics is ill health and the relief of symptoms or disease. One of the main doctrines of paediatric nursing is the notion of family focused care. Paediatric nurses work to support the family by rendering nursing care that the family cannot perform, educating and supporting them to maintain their usual caring activities and dynamically regarding the parents as partners in the care procedure. Other word for child health nursing is paediatric nursing.

Indian traditionalistic childcare practices are useful and adopted from western nursing care system like, breast-feeding and contact of a mother with the child during the hospitalization. However many child-care practices are unsafe, like, late weaning, care established on superstitions and so on. In spite of the changes in scientific technology and healthcare system, there has been small awareness to change unsafe practices. Government policies established on the World Health organization program has produced progress in preventive paediatrics extent. The national plan is to attain the objective of health for all and 100% coverage of immunization, by 2000 A.D."

This plan has developed total national health services to arrive at the roots of the society through Maternal and Child Health Services. In India, infant mortality rates are still high as compared to developed countries. As per World Health organization, Japan has the lowest infant mortality of 4 per 1,000, against India's infant mortality rate of 77 per 1,000. India's objective is to attain the infant mortality rate beneath 60 per 1,000 by the year 2,000. There is an extreme requirement for better childcare, particularly neonatal and infant care becomes very significant to attain this objective. In India, the mortality rate of under five children is reported 105 per 1,000. In Japan, it is 6 per 1,000 in 1995.

If we look at reasons of infant mortality, we detect poor socioeconomic situations and maternal ill health during pregnancy ensuing in intrauterine growth retardation and pre-maturity, spoiled obstetrical practices, and neonatal infections like diarrhoea, bronchopneumonia, and meningitis. Many a reasons of infant mortality and morbidness are avoidable.

Nurses play the crucial role in preventing infections, making better nutritional status, making better intra natal and prompt postnatal care techniques in the hospital in addition to in the society. This can be done by presentation, health education, and counselling to the parents and children for producing responsiveness and making changes toward improved healthcare practices. Healthcare of children has been noticeably changed in developed countries. There is a change in the perspective of children from "miniature adults" to "unique individuals" with unique needs and qualities. The child healthcare system should focus to meet the requirements of the children and their families by rendering complete child healthcare during the illness in addition to in health. The child healthcare is needed for promotion of health, prevention of diseases, stipulation of treatment, and follows up. Preventive measures ought to be practiced in wards, clinics, centres, and in the society, to assist the people to prevent or solve their health problems. Every nurse has her duty, in her field of work, in whatsoever capacity she works in relation to child-care.

## CONCEPT OF CHILD-CARE

The rising complexness of medical and nursing techniques has produced a need for unique field for child-care. The child-care has major importance, as the mortality and morbidity are higher in this group. Many diseases are avoidable like nutritional deficiency. The target of the paediatric nursing is to encourage the development and growth of the children and promote an optimal state of health physically, mentally, and socially, so that they may work at the peak of their capability. Because most of the responses of children are regulated by the phases of development and growth, the ages of the child is the most important reason affecting nursing activities.

For instance, fractured jaw is more distressing to an infant who is in oral phase of the development than to a child of the six years of age who has already passed this phase. The separation of the family during the hospitalization will cause an anxiety in the young child and may disturb the parent-child relationship. The nurse can minimize the psychological shock of a hospitalization experience by assisting the children to adapt to the situation instead of to suppress their feelings. Play therapy has significance in child-care, by which children can play out their problems.

To render complete care to children, the nurse must distinctly comprehend the effect of illness and hospitalization experience, upon the development and growth process of children and the effect of the developmental position of the children upon their responses to therapy. The role of the paediatric nurse has been regulated by the research findings in other health fields of prevention and therapy, in several fields of genetics, drugs, medical, and surgical techniques. It is also determined by the study carried out within the nursing profession itself.

The notion of evaluation of children is significant for rendering care to patients and their families. The work of the paediatric nurse is to encourage and support children in their adaptation process. The nurse must observe the children's health and illness state, their strengths and weaknesses, and usefulness of their dealing mechanism.

Nursing children require an improved sense of duty and improved judgment of children's health, responses, and designing for nursing management. The nurse must have patience and emotional balance while dealing with the children and their parents, specifically, in severely ill cases.

## NUTRITION IN CHILDREN

Knowledge of the nutrition in children is significant for the following:

- It helps to render most optimal nutrition to infants and children for their development and growth.
- The diet ought to be enough in calories, fluids, proteins, vitamins, and roughage. The food ought to be tasty and attractive.
- The feeding time table ought to be practiced to fulfill the children's appetite, digestibility, and necessity.
- Nutritional demands of children depend on the rate of growth of different body tissues and children's sex, age and health status.
- Evaluation of nutritional status of children is significant in total health evaluation.

Nutritional deficiency can lead to the following:

1. Growth retardation
   - i. Failure to put on weight
   - ii. Children look small for age
   - iii. Children appear thin
2. History of repeated infections
   - i. Respiratory infections
   - ii. Gastrointestinal infections
3. Symptoms associated with insufficient nutrition
   - i. Hunger, irritability, lack of concentration, exhaustion, disturbed sleep, wasting of muscles.

Healthy children are full of vitality and are active. Their development and growth are as per the expected norms and show no nutritional inadequacy. Sufficient nutrition is necessary to maintain optimal health.

## EVALUATION OF HEIGHT AND WEIGHT

Weight for along time has been used as an indicator of malnutrition. Extent of height deficit, in relation to age, points the duration of malnutrition. Weight for height is the index considered as an index of present nutritional status. The following factors ought to be regarded while evaluating the nutritional status:

- Influence of environmental situations
- Culture and habits
- Food products available
- Socioeconomic situation
- Health and educational status of parents

The child with sufficient nutrition is characterized by an erect posture, firm muscles, straight legs and spine, well-formed teeth, bright eyes, and optimal height and weight for the child's age. Poor nutritional status is characterized by sagging position, round narrow shoulders, flat chest, abdominal protuberance, curved spine, poor muscle tone, dull hair, dull eyes, knock knees, and underweight for the child's age.

## IMPORTANCE OF NUTRITION IN SICK CHILDREN

Sick children require food so that they can fight infections without using all the nutrients reserved in the body. Sick children may not feel hungry. If they eat sufficient diet, their symptoms are usually less severe than those of malnourished children. For the sick children, small frequent feeding should comprise nonirritating, easily digestible, sufficient in amount, and sufficient in quality. For instance, cereal gruels, milk, tender fish, soft cooked egg, and non-fibrous fruits, like banana may be given to the sick children.

During the recuperation, children ought to be given extra calories and proteins to make up for the inadequacy that took place during the illness.

## NUTRITION AND FEEDING - INFANT NUTRITIONAL REQUIREMENT

The neonate's immature organ system and the unparalleled growth of the early stage, of life impose unique demands for nutrients and fluids. These factors also confine the types and quantities of foods a neonate; can ingest and digest. Neonate's food must contain enough quantity of carbohydrates, proteins, fats, vitamins, minerals and fluids.

## FEEDING OF ENERGY GIVING FOOD

Three fundamental nutrients, namely carbohydrates, proteins, and fats supply the body's caloric requirements. Proteins promote cellular growth and maintenance, aid a metabolism, and contribute to many defensive substances. Fats render concentrated energy storage, transport essential nutrients (like fatty acids required for neurological development and growth), and insulate vital organs. Carbohydrate, which contain four calories per gram, should render 35% to 55% of the neonate's total calories; fats that contain nine calories per gram 30% to 55%; and proteins, which contain four calories per gram, the rest of calories.

### Vitamins and Minerals

Vitamins influence metabolic processes and promote growth and maintenance of body tissues. Fat soluble vitamins (A, D, E, and K) in excess can be stored in the body somewhat and generally are not excreted; consequently reserve, may build up. Water-soluble vitamins (C, Bl, B2, B6, B12, niacin, folic acid, pantothenic acid, and biotin) are stored only in small quantities. Therefore if these vitamins are not ingested on a regular basis, deficiencies may develop comparatively rapidly. All main minerals and trace minerals are necessary for a wide range of body functions, as well as regulation of enzyme metabolism, acid-base balance, and nerve and muscle integrity. Calcium and iron are especially significant for growth -calcium for the fast bone mineralization of the first year and for haemoglobin synthesis.

## Fluid

The neonate's difficulty in concentrating urine plus, a high extra-cellular water content result in a much greater requirement for fluid (150 ml./kg/day) as compared to the adult (20 to 30 ml./kg/day). The neonate has limited gastric capacity. Besides, fat absorption doesn't arrive at adult level till ages six to nine months. For the first month restricted splitting of the starch salivary enzyme ptyalin and deficiency of pancreatic amylase limit digestion of complex starches found in solid foods. Though the fundamental constituents of the neurological system are present at birth, myelination is incomplete. Only breast milk, infant formula and whole milk contain sufficient linoleic acid to facilitate myelination. Consequently, the milk that contains less than 2% milk fat is not suggested before age of one year.

## Breast Feeding

Human milk is believed to be perfect for a neonate. Breast milk is natural ready made food most appropriate feed for the neonate.

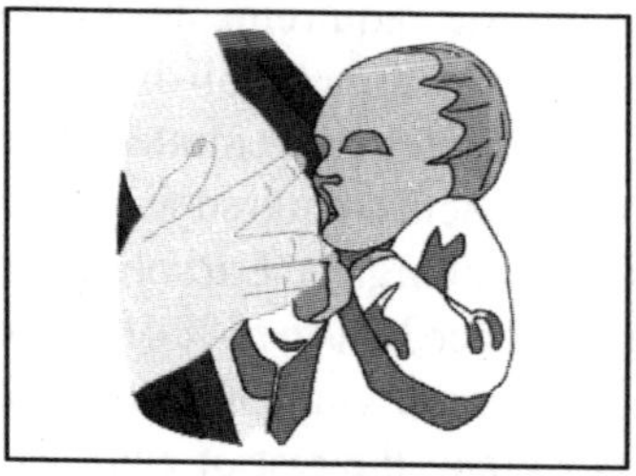

*Fig. Breast Feeding*

## Advantages of the Breast Feeding

- The breast feeding provides close physical contact between the neonate and the mother which provides satisfaction. It provides an opportunity for infant-mother attachment.
- Human milk is available at the needed temperature in needed strength and is fresh and free from contamination as it directly comes in the baby's mouth.
- Human milk contains more lacto albumin, a more comprehensive protein than casein due to its high percentage amino acids. It is more easily digested due to soft curds. Consequently, stomach emptying is fast and thus calls for frequent feeding.

- Additional lactose assists in synthesis of certain vitamins. It also contains a high quantity of crystine, an amino acid that may be necessary during the neonatal stage.
- Human milk contains higher quantity of lactose, a disaccharide, which is converted into monosaccharide glucose and galactose. Galactose is necessary for the growth of the central nervous system. Unsaturated fatty acids in the human milk assist absorption of fat and calcium in the neonate. Iron in human milk is absorbed better in the neonate.
- The human milk contains increased quantity of antibodies, immunoglobulin A (IgA), which gives immunity to the neonate against certain diseases. These antibodies are present in a high quantity in the colostrum than in mature milk. In the intestines, it acts against bacteria and viruses. Lactoferin also arrests the development of bacteria.
- It contains lacto albumin bifidus, which assist in suppressing E-coli. Lactobacillus bifidus assist to produce lactic acid, to arrest bacterial development and make the stools acidic.
- Early breast-feeding helps the mother in fast involution of the uterus and lesser chance of breast cancer.

## Antenatal Preparation

- Mothers' preparation and motivation for breast-feeding should start from the second semester of the antenatal stage. The nipple ought to be examined to see whether they are normal and protractile.
- The care of nipples is essential to prevent mechanical problems of feeding. If nipples are retracted, they ought to be pulled out at least once a day. Daily practicing, during the last trimester, can assist to prepare protractile nipples.
- The tone of the shape of the breast will be maintained by using proper brassieres.
- A diet ought to be well balanced with additional proteins, calcium, and iron.
- The mother must be persuaded that the ability to produce milk doesn't depend on the size of the breast.
- The mother ought to be told that the sufficient milk is secreted from the third day of the postpartum.

## Physiology of Lactation

Lactogen and other hormones released by the placenta and prolactin secreted by the pituitary influence the preparation of mammary glands for lactation throughout pregnancy. The breast tissues develop the glandular system, which secrete milk and encourage it to the surface of the tissue through an arrangement of alveoli and ducts. Groups of alveoli connect through milk ducts to lactiferous ducts, each conducting into lactiferous sinus, and then opening at the nipple. Each nipple receives the milk from about twenty lactiferous ducts. The alveoli starts out to secrete colostrums in mid pregnancy. At the time of the delivery, the balance between hormones changes suddenly when levels of oestrogen and progesterone decrease rapidly in absence of a placenta. Prolactin levels remain high. This change in the balance starts lactation. Most potent stimuli continue prolactin secretions are mechanical stimuli of sucking.

## HEALTH INSTRUCTIONS ON NUTRITION

Generally, people may have very small knowledge about the nutritive value. It is the duty of health workers to render suitable information to the people, in the society, hospitals, and clinics, at several levels of child development. Parents ought to be made aware of their role in practicing healthy food habits. Presentations on the preparations of simple multipurpose food can create interest in the mothers. Discussion on variety of preparations with balanced diet with the reasonable cost can assist people in daily feeding of children.

## PREVENTION OF MALNUTRITION

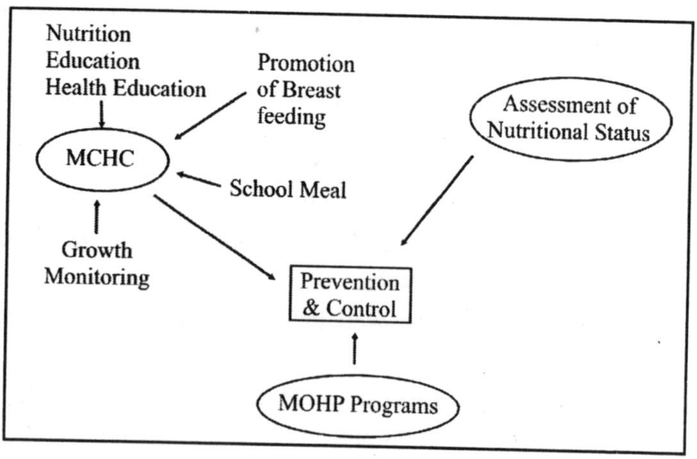


*Fig. Prevention of Malnutrition*

- The breast-feeding may be continued for six - nine months, if possible.
- Feeding diluted milk ought to be avoided.
- Weaning can be introduced from three to four months of age.
- Sufficient calories, proteins, vitamins, calcium, and iron ought to be provided to the children.
- In the early stage of diarrhoea, fever, and other diseases, the physicians or nurses' opinion may be useful.
- Spacing between children, in the family, allows better nutrition of the parenting children.
- Knowing about the cheap but nutritious origins of local food helps to select proper food.

## WEANING/INTRODUCTION TO SOLID FOODS

Weaning describes the process by which the infant progressively becomes used to the full adult diet.

## PROBLEMS DURING WEANING

- If breast-feeding is stopped, abruptly, it can have psychological and nutritional effect on the young children.
- Solid foods can cause diarrhoea, if cooked unhygienically or not digested correctly.
- If weaning foods are too poor to render sufficient nutrients, the children can develop malnutrition.

For some babies the breast-feeding may be enough for four months even though others may feel hungry even after the breast feeding and may not gain weight.

## SOLID FOODS

To begun weaning foods, the consistency of food ought to be a case increased from liquid to semi-solid and then, from semi-solid to solid foods. It is advisable to begun one or two spoons of the new food at first.

It ought to be given when a child is hungry, just before the regular feeding during the daytime. It may be continued for a few days till the child gets used to the same. Then the new food item may be commenced, one af a time. Always, the fresh food ought to be given. The quantity ought to be increased a case. The child should never be forced to eat.

Children may spit out initially. As children like to participate in feeding, their hands ought to be washed. Those who feed the child must wash their hands. Clean utensils must be used to prepare the food. The food should be, always, covered. The solids should he fed a case, on a regular basis, as per children's likes. Children ought to be observed for an indigestion, abdominal pain, diarrhoea, or rash, because some children may be allergic to certain food. Such problems associated with feeding, ought to be reported to the physician.

## CHOOSING OF WEANING FOODS

A food chosen for the weaning ought to be appropriate to the family. It ought to be easily available, low in cost, and used often in most households. The local methods of food preparation may be advised. Cooking methods that use minimum fuel and less time ought to be suggested. Rules of food hygiene ought to be followed to prevent infections. By the age of one year, the infant can eat solid foods. The child can eat with the family. For the infants and children, the volume of the, meal shouldn't be large. The child can eat two hundred ml. of foods at a time. If children are eating only three small meals a day, one of those must have high concentrated calories and proteins to meet their requirements for 24 hours.

## WEANING FOODS

Following are the cases of weaning foods that may be commenced as per child's ability to feed.

Liquids: Soup of vegetables, tomato, pulses (daals) and fruit juices.

Semi-solids food: Potato, pulses, and root vegetables can be well prepared and mashed before feeding. A banana can be mashed and fed. Soft cooked rice and soft cooked fish can be mashed before feeding. To increase the nutritive value, preparations can be used, like, ragi + jaggary. Bengal gram (Chana) powder + jaggary + ghee + sugar will supply proteins, calories, and iron.

Solid foods: Cooked rice, chapatti, idali, bread, biscuits, groundnuts, roasted chana, and banana. Solid food can be commenced when the children learn to chew correctly.

# IMMUNIZATION IN CHILDREN

The significant aspect in the childcare, is to protect children against specific preventable diseases. There are a few common dangerous infections in the childhood which are preventable by immunization, like, poliomyelitis, diphtheria, pertussis, measles, rubella, and hepatitis B. The immunizations against these diseases induce the child's body to produce immunity against particular infections. The children with malnutrition have low resistance to fight against the infections, consequently, children require timely immunization. All children have a right to get vaccines, protection against preventable diseases. Extremely malnourished children may show severe reaction to certain vaccines because they have low antibodies. For instance, measles vaccine. Immunization ought to be done with potent immunising agents to have expected results. These immunising agents may be as following:

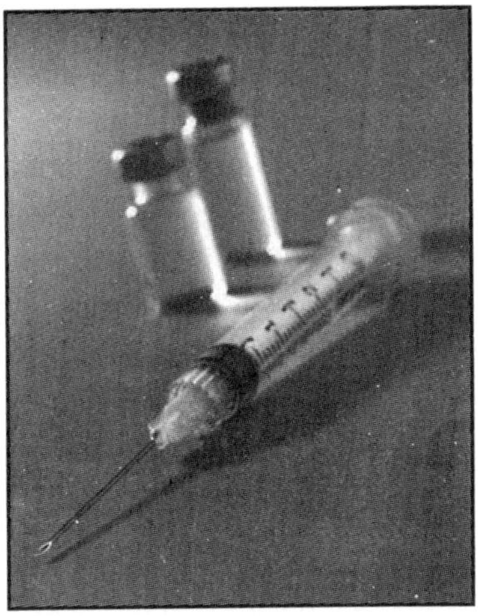

*Fig. Immunization in Children*

- Killed suspension. For instance, cholera vaccine.
- Live attenuated vaccines. For instance. Measles,
- Mumps, and Rubella (MMR) vaccines
- Toxoid. For instance, Tetanus toxoid.

## MAINTAINING A COLD CHAIN

It is necessary to preserve the favourable temperature, with cold storage, to preserve the potency of vaccines. The temperature ought to be around 2°C to 8°C. The vaccines ought to be kept under me freezing compartment. The thermometer ought to be placed in the freeze to confirm the validity. The door of the refrigerator ought to be opened as minimum as possible. During the transportation, the vaccines ought to be kept in a container maintaining the cited temperature or may be kept in a plastic bag in the icebox. The vaccines ought to be arranged as per their expiry dates for the improved use.

## CONTRAINDICATIONS FOR THE IMMUNIZATION

1. An acute illness with fever.
2. When the child is on immuno-suppresive drugs or on radiation.
3. A child suffering from leukemia, lymphoma or malignancy.

## PRECAUTIONS

Immunization with live vaccines shouldn't be repeated before three weeks. A special care ought to be taken as advised for particular vaccination as follows:

B.C.G. Vaccine: B.C.G. vaccine is prepared in a powder form and can be stored for six months. Before the use, it is dissolved with Door Closer normal saline. After dissolving it is used within twenty-four hours. The common dose is 0.1 ml. It is given on the left upper arm, intra dermal. Two to three weeks after the vaccination, a papule appears. It may heal and a scar may be formed. Parents ought to be instructed not to put anything on the site on injection.

Polio Vaccine: Oral polio vaccine is prepared with the three types of live attenuated polio viruses. Potency of this vaccine ought to be maintained by the cold chain. Three doses are given. The gap between two consequent doses ought to be four to six weeks.

It is desirable to instruct the parents not to give anything by mouth, to the child about half-hour before and after giving the polio vaccine. It is essential to give polio vaccine to those children who have suffered from the poliomyelitis, to protect them from the other two viruses, against which they may not have immunity.

Diphtheria, Pertussis and Tetanus Vaccine (DPT): DPT. Vaccine contains toxoid of diphtheria and Tetanus bacilli and dead bacilli of pertussis. It ought to be used within ten days if kept at the room temperature. The usual dose is 0.5 ml. It is given deep intramuscularly. The site for administration for the infants is best at upper and outer middle one third of the thigh.

Typhoid Vaccine: It is prepared with salmonella typhi and organism of paratyphoid A and B. It is given during the epidemic. The usual dose of administration is 0.5 ml. and 1.0 ml. subcutaneously, at the gap of 7 to 10 days.

Cholera Vaccine: It is prepared in a saline suspension of killed vibrio cholera. It is given in two doses of 0.5 ml. and 1.0 ml. epidermal at the gap of three weeks.

## THE ROLE OF A PAEDIATRIC NURSE

Wherever paediatric nurses practice, their major work is the welfare of the child and his family. In this country, because of a dearth of paediatric nurses, even fully trained nurses, the home care of the child is dealt with by society health worker or auxiliary nurses.

Nursing of the children is targeted at the highest possible state of health to each child. It includes preventing diseases or injuries, assisting children to meet their health requirements, to attain and preserve sufficient health and development, and rehabilitating them, who have deviated from usual routine. The role of the paediatric nurse depends on her education, experience, job structure, and professional requirements.

### Preventive Care

Prevention of illness and injury is significant in the role of the paediatric nurse. Preventive care ought to be regarded in relation to all aspects of the children's health. The nurse must plan care for even-aspect of development and growth of the child. Problems associated with development, nutrition, immunization, dental care, safety, socialisation, and education ought to be assessed. Any needed counselling ought to be provided.

### Health Education

The nurse should give suitable health teaching with normal feedback from the parents. She should give health instructions, as planned talks or incidental teaching as needed. The nurse can act as a model for the parents and children by her manners and behaviours.

### Restoration of Health

The nurses' role in the restoration of health is accomplished through care giving activities. While nursing the sick children, the nurse is involved in meeting their requirements like feeding, bathing, security, comfort, and other care. She must do continual evaluation and assessment, to modify the care plan and meet the developmental requirements, which regulate children's health. The rehabilitation of physically or mentally disabled children is also a significant aspect of restoration.

## Coordination

The nurse plays a significant role in the health team by coordinating activities associated with patient care, which are interdependent on several health team workers and departments.

The communication and coordination may be direct or indirect, depending upon healthcare system. In short, the paediatric nurse can render complete care, to the infants and children including counselling to the parents, about their role in the child-care.

## REFERENCES

Rudolph MC, Levene MI. Paediatrics and child health. Oxford: Blackwell Science; 1999.

Rudy C. Developmental dysplasia of the hip: what's new in the 1990's. J Pediatr Health Care 1996; 10(2):85.

Thomas DO. Assessing children—it's different. RN 1996; 59(4):38-44.

Unti SM. The critical first year of life: history, physical examination and general developmental assessment. Pediatr Clin North Am 1994; 41(5):859-873.

Vessey JA. Developmental approaches to examining young children. Pediatr Nurs 1995;21(l):53-56.

Wong DL. The paper doll technique. Pediatr Nurs 1981; 7:39-40.

Wong DL, Wilson D. Whaley and Wong's nursing care of infants and children, 6th edn. St. Louis: Mosby; 1999.

# 2

# Modern Concepts of Childcare

## INTERNATIONALLY ACCEPTED RIGHTS OF THE CHILD

Understanding that the child, for the total and harmonious evolution of his or her personality, should grow up in a family atmosphere, in an atmosphere of happiness, love and understanding.

Considering that the child ought to be fully prepared to live a personal life in society, and brought up in the spirit of the ideals proclaimed in the Charter of the United Nations, and particularly in the spirit of peace, dignity, tolerance, freedom, equality and solidarity.

Taking into account that the need to extend specific care to the child has been stated in the Geneva Declaration of the Rights of the Child of 1924 and in the Declaration of the Rights of the Child adopted by the General Assembly on twenty November 1959 and recognized in the Universal Declaration of Human Rights, in the International Covenant on Civil and Political Rights (particularly in articles twenty-three and twenty-four), in the International Covenant on Economic, Social and Cultural Rights (particularly in article ten) and in the statutes and relevant instruments of specialized agencies and international organizations concerned with the welfare of children.

Taking into account that, as indicated in the Declaration of the Rights of the Child, "the child, by reason of his physical and mental immaturity, requires exceptional safeguards and care, including suitable legal protection, before in addition to after birth".

Remembering the provisions of the Declaration on Social and Legal Principles pertaining to the Protection and Welfare of Children, with Special Reference to Foster Placement and Adoption Nationally and Internationally; the United Nations Standard Minimum Rules for the Administration of

Juvenile Justice; and the Declaration on the Protection of Women and Children in Emergency and Armed Conflict, Recognizing that, in all countries in the world, there are children living in exceptionally difficult situations, and that such children need special consideration.

Taking due account of the importance of the traditions and cultural values of each people for the protection and harmonious development of the child,

Recognizing the importance of international co-operation for making better the living situations of children in every country, particularly in the developing countries,

Have agreed as follows:

## PART I

### Article 1

- A child means every human being beneath the age of eighteen years unless under the law applicable to the child, majority is achieved earlier.

### Article 2

- States Parties shall respect and ensure the rights set forth in the present Convention to each child within their jurisdiction without discrimination of any kind, irrespective of the child's or his or her parent's or legal guardian's race, colour, sex, language, religion, political or other opinion, national, ethnic or social origin, property, disability, birth or other status.
- States Parties shall take all suitable measures to ensure that the child is protected against all forms of discrimination or punishment on the basis of the status, activities, expressed opinions, or beliefs of the child's parents, legal guardians, or family members.

### Article 3

- In all actions concerning children, whether undertaken by public or private social welfare institutions, courts of law, administrative authorities or legislative bodies, the best interests of the child shall be a primary consideration.
- States Parties undertake to ensure the child such protection and care as is essential for his or her well-being, taking into account the rights and responsibilities of his or her parents,

legal guardians, or other individuals legally responsible for him or her, and, to this end, shall take all suitable legislative and administrative measures.

- States Parties shall ensure that the institutions, services and facilities responsible for the care or protection of children shall conform with the standards established by competent authorities, especially in the fields of safety, health, in the number and suitability of their staff, in addition to competent supervision.

**Article 4**

- States Parties shall undertake all suitable legislative, administrative, and other measures for the implementation of the rights recognized in the present Convention. With regard to economic, social and cultural rights, States Parties shall undertake such measures to the maximum extent of their available resources and, where required, within the framework of international co-operation.

**Article 5**

- States Parties shall respect the duties, rights and responsibilities of parents or, where applicable, the members of the extended family or society as provided for by local custom, legal guardians or other persons legally responsible for the child, to render, in a manner consistent with the evolving capacities of the child, suitable direction and guidance in the exercise by the child of the rights recognized in the present Convention.

**Article 6**

- States Parties recognize that every child has the inherent right to life.
- States Parties shall ensure to the maximum extent possible the survival and development of the child.

**Article 7**

- The child shall be registered promptly after birth and shall have the right from birth to a name, the right to acquire a nationality and. as far as possible, the right to know and be cared for by his or her parents.
- States Parties shall ensure the implementation of these rights in accordance with their national law and their obligations under

the relevant international instruments in this field, particularly where the child would otherwise be stateless.

**Article 8**

- States Parties undertake to respect the right of the child to preserve his or her identity, including nationality, name and family relations as recognized by law without unlawful interference.
- Where a child is illegally deprived of some or all of the elements of his or her identity, States Parties shall render suitable assistance and protection, with a view to re-establishing speedily his or her identity.

**Article 9**

- States Parties shall ensure that a child shall not be separated from his or her parents against their will, except when competent authorities subject to judicial review determine, in accordance with applicable law and procedures, that such separation is essential for the best interests of the child. Such determination may be essential in a specific case like one involving abuse or neglect of the child by the parents, or one where the parents are living separately and a decision must be made as to the child's place of residence.
- In any proceedings pursuant to paragraph one of the present article, all interested parties shall be given an opportunity to participate in the proceedings and make their views known.
- States Parties shall respect the right of the child who is separated from one or both parents to preserve individual relations and direct contact with both parents on a regular basis, except if it is contrary to the child's best interests.
- Where such separation results from any action started by a State Party, like the detention, imprisonment, exile, deportation or death (including death arising from any cause while the person is in the custody of the State) of one or both parents or of the child, that State Party shall, upon request, render the parents, the child or, if suitable, other member of the family with the necessary information concerning the whereabouts of the absent member(s) of the family unless the provision of the information would be detrimental to the well-being of the child. States Parties shall further ensure that the submission of

such a request shall of itself entail no adverse consequences for the person(s) concerned.

**Article 10**

- In accordance with the obligation of States Parties under article 9, paragraph one, applications by a child or his or her parents to enter or leave a State Party for the intention of family reunification shall be dealt with by States Parties in a positive, humane and expeditious manner. States Parties shall further ensure that the submission of such a request shall entail no adverse consequences for the applicants and for the members of their family.
- A child whose parents reside in different States shall have the right to preserve on a regular basis, save in exceptional circumstances personal relations and direct contacts with both parents. Towards that end and in accordance with the obligation of States Parties under article 9, paragraph one, States Parties shall respect the right of the child and his or her parents to leave any country, including their own, and to enter their own country. The right to leave any country shall be subject only to such restrictions as are prescribed by law and which are essential to protect the national security, public order (ordre public), public health or morals or the rights and freedoms of others and are consistent with the other rights recognized in the present Convention.

**Article 11**

- States Parties shall take measures to combat the illicit transfer and non-return of children abroad.
- To this end, States Parties shall promote the conclusion of bilateral or multilateral agreements or accession to existing agreements.

**Article 12**

- States Parties shall assure to the child who is capable of forming his or her own views the right to express those views freely in all matters affecting the child, the views of the child being given due weight in accordance with the age and maturity of the child.
- For this intention, the child shall particularly be provided the opportunity to be heard in any judicial and administrative

proceedings affecting the child, either directly, or through a representative or a suitable body, in a manner consistent with the procedural rules of national law.

**Article 13**

- The child shall have the right to freedom of expression; this right shall include freedom to seek, receive and impart information and concepts of all kinds, regardless of frontiers, either orally, in writing or in print, in the form of art, or through any other media of the child's choice.
- The exercise of this right may be subject to certain restrictions, but these shall only be like are provided by law and are essential:
  - For respect of the rights or reputations of others; or
  - For the protection of national security or of public order (ordre public), or of public health or morals.

**Article 14**

- States Parties shall respect the right of the child to freedom of thought, conscience and religion.
- States Parties shall respect the rights and responsibilities of the parents and, when applicable, legal guardians, to render direction to the child in the exercise of his or her right in a manner consistent with the evolving capacities of the child.
- Freedom to manifest one's religion or beliefs may be subject only to such limitations as are prescribed by law and are essential to protect public safety, order, health or morals, or the fundamental rights and freedoms of others.

**Article 15**

- States Parties recognize the rights of the child to freedom of association and to freedom of peaceful assembly.
- No restrictions may be placed on the exercise of these rights other than those imposed in conformity with the law and which are essential in a democratic society in the interests of national security or public safety, public order (ordre public), the protection of public health or morals or the protection of the rights and freedoms of others.

**Article 16**

- No child shall be subjected to arbitrary or unlawful interference with his or her privacy, family, home or correspondence, nor to unlawful attacks on his or her honour and reputation.

- The child has the right to the protection of the law against such interference or attacks.

**Article 17**

- States Parties recognize the significant work performed by the mass media and shall ensure that the child has access to information and material from a diversity of national and international sources, particularly those targeted at the promotion of his or her social, spiritual and moral well-being and physical and mental health. To this end, States Parties shall:
  - Encourage the mass media to disseminate information and material of social and cultural benefit to the child and in accordance with the spirit of article 29;
  - Encourage international co-operation in the production, exchange and dissemination of such information and material from a diversity of cultural, national and international sources;
  - Encourage the production and dissemination of children's books;
  - Encourage the mass media to have specific regard to the linguistic requirements of the child who belongs to a minority group or who is indigenous;
  - Encourage the development of suitable guidelines for the protection of the child from information and material injurious to his or her well-being, bearing in mind the provisions of articles 13 and 18.

**Article 18**

- States Parties shall use their best efforts to ensure recognition of the principle that both parents have common duties for the upbringing and development of the child. Parents or, as the case may be, legal guardians, have the primary duty for the upbringing and development of the child. The best interests of the child will be their fundamental concern.
- For the intention of guaranteeing and promoting the rights set forth in the present Convention, States Parties shall provide suitable assistance to parents and legal guardians in the performance of their child-rearing duties and shall ensure the development of institutions, facilities and services for the care of children.

- States Parties shall take all suitable measures to ensure that children of working parents have the right to benefit from child-care services and facilities for which they are eligible.

**Article 19**

- States Parties shall take all suitable legislative, administrative, social and educational measures to protect the child from all forms of physical or mental violence, injury or abuse, neglect or negligent treatment, maltreatment or exploitation, including sexual abuse, while in the care of parent(s), legal guardian(s) or any other person who has the care of the child.
- Such protective measures should, as suitable, include effective procedures for the establishment of social programmes to render essential support for the child and for those who have the care of the child, in addition to for other forms of prevention and for identification, reporting, referral, investigation, treatment and follow-up of instances of child maltreatment described heretofore, and, as suitable, for judicial involvement.

**Article 20**

- A child temporarily or permanently deprived of his or her family environment, or in whose own best interests can't be allowed to remain in that environment, shall be entitled to special protection and assistance provided by the State.
- States Parties shall in accordance with their national laws ensure alternative care for such a child.
- Such care could include, inter alia, foster placement, kafalah of Islamic law, adoption or if essential placement in appropriate institutions for the care of children. When considering solutions, due regard shall be paid to the desirability of continuity in a child's upbringing and to the child's ethnic, religious, cultural and linguistic background.

**Article 21**

- States Parties that recognize and/or permit the system of adoption shall ensure that the best interests of the child shall be the paramount consideration and they shall:
- Ensure that the adoption of a child is authorized only by competent authorities who determine, in accordance with applicable law and procedures and on the basis of all pertinent

and reliable information, that the adoption is permissible in view of the child's status concerning parents, relatives and legal guardians and that, if needed, the persons concerned have given their informed consent to the adoption on the basis of such counselling as may be essential;

— Recognize that inter-country adoption may be regarded as an alternative means of child's care, if the child can't be placed in a foster or an adoptive family or can't in any appropriate manner be cared for in the child's country of origin; (c) Ensure that the child concerned by inter-country adoption enjoys safeguards and standards equivalent to those existing in the case of national adoption;

— Take all suitable measures to ensure that, in inter-country adoption, the placement doesn't result in improper financial gain for those involved in it;

— Promote, where suitable, the objectives of the present article by concluding bilateral or multilateral arrangements or agreements, and endeavour, within this framework, to ensure that the placement of the child in another country is carried out by competent authorities or organs.

**Article 22**

- States Parties shall take suitable measures to ensure that a child who is seeking refugee status or who is believed to be a refugee in accordance with applicable international or domestic law and procedures shall, whether unaccompanied or accompanied by his or her parents or by any other person, receive suitable protection and humanitarian assistance in the enjoyment of applicable rights set forth in the present Convention and in other international human rights or humanitarian instruments to which the said States are Parties.

- For this intention, States Parties shall render, as they consider suitable, co-operation in any efforts by the United Nations and other competent intergovernmental organizations or non-governmental organizations co-operating with the United Nations to protect and assist such a child and to trace the parents or other members of the family of any refugee child in order to obtain information essential for reunification with his or her family. In cases where no parents or other members of the family can be found, the child shall be accorded the same protection as any other child permanently or temporarily deprived of his or her family environment for any reason, as set forth in the present Convention.

**Article 23**

- States Parties recognize that a mentally or physically disabled child should enjoy a full and decent life, in situations which ensure dignity, promote self-reliance and facilitate the child's active participation in the society.
- States Parties recognize the right of the disabled child to unique care and shall encourage and ensure the extension, subject to available resources, to the eligible child and those responsible for his or her care, of assistance for which application is made and which is suitable to the child's condition and to the circumstances of the parents or others caring for the child. 3. Recognizing the unique requirements of a disabled child, assistance extended in accordance with paragraph 2 of the present article shall be provided free of charge, whenever possible, taking into account the financial resources of the parents or others caring for the child, and shall be designed to ensure that the disabled child has effective access to and receives education, training, healthcare services, rehabilitation services, preparation for employment and recreation opportunities in a manner conducive to the child's achieving the fullest possible social integration and personal development, including his or her cultural and spiritual development
- States Parties shall promote, in the spirit of international cooperation, the exchange of suitable information in the field of preventive healthcare and of medical, psychological and functional treatment of disabled children, including dissemination of and access to information concerning methods of rehabilitation, education and vocational services, with the target of enabling States Parties to improve their capabilities and skills and to widen their experience in these fields. In this regard, specific account shall be taken of the requirements of developing countries.

**Article 24**

- States Parties recognize the right of the child to the enjoyment of the highest attainable standard of health and to facilities for the treatment of illness and rehabilitation of health. States Parties shall strive to ensure that no child is deprived of his or her right of access to such healthcare services.

- States Parties shall pursue full implementation of this right and, particularly, shall take suitable measures:
  - To diminish infant and child mortality;
  - To ensure the provision of essential medical assistance and healthcare to all children with emphasis on the development of primary health care;
  - To combat disease and malnutrition, including within the framework of primary health care, through, inter alia, the application of readily available technology and through the provision of sufficient nutritious foods and clean drinking-water, taking into consideration the dangers and risks of environmental pollution;
  - To ensure suitable pre-natal and post-natal healthcare for mothers;
  - To ensure that all segments of society, particularly parents and children, are informed, have access to education and are supported in the use of fundamental knowledge of child health and nutrition, the advantages of breastfeeding, hygiene and environmental sanitation and the prevention of accidents;
  - To develop preventive health care, counselling for parents and family planning education and services.
- States Parties shall take all effective and suitable measures with a view to abolishing traditional practices prejudicial to the health of children.
- States Parties undertake to promote and encourage international co-operation with a view to achieving progressively the full realization of the right recognized in the present article. In this regard, specific account shall be taken of the requirements of developing countries.

**Article 25**

- States Parties recognize the right of a child who has been placed by the competent authorities for the intentions of care, protection or treatment of his or her physical or mental health, to a periodic review of the treatment provided to the child and all other circumstances relevant to his or her placement.

**Article 26**

- States Parties shall recognize for every child the right to benefit from social security, including social insurance, and shall take the essential measures to attain the full realization of this right in accordance with their national law.
- The benefits should, where suitable, be granted, taking into account the resources and the circumstances of the child and persons having duty for the maintenance of the child, in addition to any other consideration relevant to an application for benefits made by or on behalf of the child.

**Article 27**

- States Parties recognize the right of every child to a standard of living sufficient for the child's physical, mental, spiritual, moral and social development.
- The parent(s) or others responsible for the child have the primary duty to secure, within their abilities and financial capacities, the conditions of living essential for the child's development.
- States Parties, in accordance with national conditions and within their means, shall take suitable measures to assist parents and others responsible for the child to implement this right and shall in case of need render material assistance and support programmes, especially with regard to nutrition, clothing and housing.
- States Parties shall take all suitable measures to secure the recuperation or maintenance for the child from the parents or other persons having financial duty for the child, both within the State Party and from abroad. Particularly, where the person having financial duty for the child lives in a State different from that of the child, States Parties shall promote the accession to international agreements or the conclusion of such agreements, in addition to the making of other suitable arrangements.

**Article 28**

- States Parties recognize the right of the child to education, and with a view to achieving this right progressively and on the basis of equal opportunity, they shall, particularly:
  - Make primary education compulsory and available free to all;

— Encourage the development of different forms of secondary education, including normal and vocational education, make them available and accessible to every child, and take suitable measures like the introduction of free education and offering financial assistance in case of need;
— Make higher education accessible to all on the basis of capacity by every suitable means;
— Make educational and vocational information and counselling available and accessible to all children;
— Take measures to encourage regular attendance at schools and the reduction of drop-out rates.

- States Parties shall take all suitable measures to ensure that school discipline is administered in a manner consistent with the child's human dignity and in conformity with the present Convention.
- States Parties shall promote and encourage international cooperation in matters relating to education, particularly with a view to contributing to the elimination of ignorance and illiteracy all through the world and facilitating access to scientific and technical knowledge and modern teaching methods. In this regard, particular account shall be taken of the needs of developing countries.

**Article 29**

General Comment on its Implementation:

States Parties agree that the education of the child shall be directed to:

- The development of the child's personality, talents and mental and physical abilities to their fullest potential;
- The development of respect for human rights and fundamental freedoms, and for the principles enshrined in the Charter of the United Nations;
- The development of respect for the child's parents, his or her own cultural identity, language and values, for the national values of the country in which the child is living, the country from which he or she may originate, and for civilizations different from his or her own;

- The preparation of the child for responsible life in a free society, in the spirit of understanding, peace, tolerance, equality of sexes, and friendship amongst all peoples, ethnic, national and religious groups and persons of indigenous origin;
- The development of respect for the natural environment.
- No part of the present article or article 28 shall be construed so as to interfere with the liberty of individuals and bodies to establish and direct educational institutions, subject always to the observance of the principle set forth in paragraph one of the present article and to the requirements that the education given in such institutions shall conform to such minimum standards as may be laid down by the State.

**Article 30**

- In those States in which ethnic, religious or linguistic minorities or persons of indigenous origin exist, a child belonging to such a minority or who is indigenous shall not be denied the right, in society with other members of his or her group, to enjoy his or her own culture, to profess and practise his or her own religion, or to use his or her own language.

**Article 31**

- States Parties recognize the right of the child to rest and leisure, to engage in play and recreational activities suitable to the age of the child and to participate freely in cultural life and the arts.
- States Parties shall respect and promote the right of the child to participate fully in cultural and artistic life and shall encourage the provision of suitable and equal opportunities for cultural, artistic, recreational and leisure activity.

**Article 32**

- States Parties recognize the right of the child to be protected from economic exploitation and from performing any work that is likely to be hazardous or to interfere with the child's education, or to be unsafe to the child's health or physical, mental, spiritual, moral or social development.
- States Parties shall take legislative, administrative, social and educational measures to ensure the implementation of the present article. To this end, and having regard to the relevant

provisions of other international instruments, States Parties shall particularly:

— Render for a minimum age or minimum ages for admission to employment;
— Render for suitable regulation of the hours and conditions of employment;
— Render for suitable penalties or other sanctions to ensure the effective enforcement of the present article.

**Article 33**

- States Parties shall take all suitable measures, including legislative, administrative, social and educational measures, to protect children from the illicit use of narcotic drugs and psychotropic substances as defined in the relevant international treaties, and to prevent the use of children in the illicit production and trafficking of such substances.

**Article 34**

- States Parties undertake to protect the child from all forms of sexual exploitation and sexual abuse. For these intentions, States Parties shall particularly take all suitable national, bilateral and multilateral measures to prevent:
  — The inducement or coercion of a child to engage in any unlawful sexual activity;
  — The exploitative use of children in prostitution or other unlawful sexual practices;
  — The exploitative use of children in pornographic performances and materials.

**Article 35**

- States Parties shall take all suitable national, bilateral and multilateral measures to prevent the abduction of, the sale of or traffic in children for any intention or in any form.

**Article 36**

- States Parties shall protect the child against all other forms of exploitation prejudicial to any aspects of the child's welfare.

**Article 37**

States Parties shall ensure that:

- No child shall be subjected to torture or other cruel, inhuman or degrading treatment or punishment. Neither capital punishment nor life imprisonment without possibility of release shall be imposed for offences committed by persons beneath eighteen years of age;

- No child shall be deprived of his or her liberty unlawfully or arbitrarily. The arrest, detention or imprisonment of a child shall be in conformity with the law and shall be used only as a measure of last resort and for the shortest suitable stage of time;
- Every child deprived of liberty shall be treated with humanity and respect for the inherent dignity of the human person, and in a manner which takes into account the needs of persons of his or her age. Particularly, every child deprived of liberty shall be separated from adults unless it is believed to be in the child's best interest not to do so and shall have the right to preserve contact with his or her family through correspondence and visits, save in exceptional circumstances;
- Every child deprived of his or her liberty shall have the right to prompt access to legal and other suitable assistance, in addition to the right to challenge the legality of the deprivation of his or her liberty before a court or other competent, independent and impartial authority, and to a prompt decision on any such action.

**Article 38**

- States Parties undertake to respect and to ensure respect for rules of international humanitarian law applicable to them in armed conflicts which are relevant to the child.
- States Parties shall take all feasible measures to ensure that persons who have not achieved the age of fifteen years don't take a direct part in hostilities.
- States Parties shall refrain from recruiting any person who has not achieved the age of fifteen years into their armed forces. In recruiting amongst those persons who have achieved the age of fifteen years but who have not achieved the age of eighteen years, States Parties shall endeavour to give priority to those who are oldest.
- In accordance with their obligations under international humanitarian law to protect the civilian population in armed conflicts, States Parties shall take all feasible measures to ensure

protection and care of children who are affected by an armed conflict.

**Article 39**

- States Parties shall take all suitable measures to promote physical and psychological recuperation and social reintegration of a child victim of: any form of neglect, exploitation, or abuse; torture or any other form of cruel, inhuman or degrading treatment or punishment; or armed conflicts. Such recuperation and reintegration shall take place in an environment which encourages the health, self-respect and dignity of the child.

**Article 40**

- States Parties recognize the right of every child alleged as, accused of, or recognized as having infringed the penal law to be treated in a manner consistent with the promotion of the child's sense of dignity and worth, which reinforces the child's respect for the human rights and fundamental freedoms of others and which takes into account the child's age and the desirability of promoting the child's reintegration and the child's assuming a constructive role in society.
- To this end, and having regard to the relevant provisions of international instruments, States Parties shall, particularly, ensure that:
    - No child shall be alleged as, be accused of, or recognized as having infringed the penal law by reason of acts or omissions that were not prohibited by national or international law at the time they were committed;
    - Every child alleged as or accused of having infringed the penal law has at least the following guarantees:
        - To be presumed innocent till proven guilty as per law;
        - To be informed promptly and directly of the charges against him or her, and, if suitable, through his or her parents or legal guardians, and to have legal or other suitable assistance in the preparation and demonstration of his or her defence;
        - To have the matter determined without delay by a competent, independent and impartial authority or judicial body in a fair hearing as per law, in the presence of legal or other suitable assistance and, unless it is regarded not

to be in the best interest of the child, particularly, taking into account his or her age or situation, his or her parents or legal guardians;

- Not to be compelled to give testimony or to confess guilt; to examine or have examined adverse witnesses and to obtain the participation and examination of witnesses on his or her behalf under conditions of equality;
- If regarded to have infringed the penal law, to have this decision and any measures imposed in consequence thereof reviewed by a higher competent, independent and impartial authority or judicial body as per law;
- To have the free assistance of an interpreter if the child can't understand or speak the language used;
- To have his or her privacy fully respected at all stages of the proceedings. 3. States Parties shall seek to promote the establishment of laws, procedures, authorities and institutions specially applicable to children alleged as, accused of, or recognized as having infringed the penal law, and, particularly:

— The establishment of a minimum age beneath which children shall be presumed not to have the capacity to infringe the penal law;

— Whenever suitable and desirable, measures for dealing with such children without resorting to judicial proceedings, rendering that human rights and legal safeguards are fully respected.

- A variety of dispositions, like care, counselling and supervision orders; counselling; probation; foster care; education and vocational training programmes and other alternatives to institutional care shall be available to ensure that children are dealt with in a manner suitable to their well-being and proportionate both to their circumstances and the offence.

**Article 41**

Nothing in the present Convention shall affect any provisions which are more conducive to the realization of the rights of the child and which may be contained in:

- The law of a State party; or
- International law in force for that State.

## NATIONAL POLICY AND LEGISLATIONS FOR CHILD HEALTH AND WELFARE

There are several constitutional provisions for children. These include the following.

- Article 14 provides that the State shall not deny to any person equality before the law or the equal protection of the laws within the territory of India.
- Article 15(3) provides that, "Nothing in this article shall prevent the State for making any unique provision for women and children."
- Article 21 render that no person shall be deprived of his life or personal liberty except as per procedure established by law.
- Article 21A directs the State shall render free and compulsory education to all children of the age of six to fourteen years in such manner as the State may, by law, determine.
- Article 23 prohibits trafficking of human beings and forced labour.
- Article 24 prohibits employment of children beneath the age of fourteen years in factories, mines or any other hazardous occupation.
- Article 25-28 provides freedom of conscience, and free profession, practice and propagation of religion.
- Article 39(e) and (f) render that the State shall, particularly, direct its policy towards securing to ensure that the health and strength of workers, men and women and the tender age of children are not abused and that the citizens are not forced by economic necessity to enter avocations unsuited to their age or strength and that the children are given opportunities and facilities to develop in a healthy manner and in conditions of freedom and dignity and that the childhood and the parents are protected against exploitation and against moral and material abandonment.
- Article 45 envisages that the State shall endeavour to render early childhood care and education for all children till they complete the age of six years.

## LEGISLATIONS

There are several Legislations pertaining to children. These include the following.

- The Child Marriage Restraint Act, 1929.
- The Child Labour (Prohibition and Regulation) Act, 1986.
- The Juvenile Justice (Care and Protection of Children) Act, 2000.
- The Infant Milk Substitutes, Feeding Bottles and Infant Foods (Regulation of Production, Supply and Distribution) Act, 1992.
- The Pre-Conception and Pre-natal Diagnostic Technique (Prohibition of Sex Selection) Act, 1994.
- The Persons with Disabilities (Equal Opportunities, Protection of Rights and Full Participation) Act, 1995.
- The Immoral Traffic (Prevention) Act, 1956.
- The Guardian and Wards Act, 1890.
- The young Persons (Harmful Publications) Act, 1956.
- The Commissions for Protection of Child Rights Act, 2005

## POLICIES

The National Policy for Children was adopted on 22nd Aug., 1974. This Policy lays down that the State shall render sufficient services towards children, both before and after birth and during the growing stages for their full physical, mental and social development. The measures recommended include amongst others, a complete health programme, supplementary nutrition for mothers and children, free and compulsory education for all children up to the age of 14 years, promotion of physical education and recreational activities, unique consideration for children of weaker sections such as SCs and STs, prevention of exploitation of children, etc.

The Government of India adopted the National Charter for Children which has been prepared after obtaining the views/comments and suggestions of the State Governments/UT Administrations, concerned Ministries and Departments and experts in the field. The National Charter is a statement of intent embodying the Government's agenda for Children. The document emphasizes Government of India's commitment to children's rights to survival, health and nutrition, standard of living, play and leisure, early childhood care, education, protection of the girl child, empowering adolescents, equality, life and liberty, name and nationality, freedom of expression, freedom of association and peaceful assembly, the right to a family and the right to be protected from economic exploitation and all forms of abuse. It also provides for protection of children in difficult circumstances, children with disabilities, children from marginalised and disadvantaged communities, and child victims. The document while stipulating the responsibilities of the State and the Society towards children also emphasizes the responsibilities of children towards family, society and the Nation. The National Charter for Children was notified in the Gazette of India on 9th Feb., 2004.

India acceded to the UN Convention on the Rights of the Child on 11th Dec., 1992 to reiterate its commitment to the cause of children. The target of the Convention is to give every child the right to survival and development in a healthy and congenial environment.

India is also party to the Millennium Development Goals and the SAARC Conventions on Child Welfare and Combating Trafficking of Women and Children in SAARC Region.

National Plan of Action for Children 2005 M/o of Women and Child Development has prepared a National Plan of Action for Children 2005 after harmonizing the targets for children set in the UN General Assembly Special Session on Children held in 2002 and the monitorable targets set in the Tenth Five Year Plan, and targets for children in related Ministries/ Departments. The Action Plan has been prepared in consultation with concerned Ministries and Departments, States/Union territory Governments, Non Governmental Organizations and experts. The National Plan of Action includes targets, objectives, strategies and activities for making better nutritional status of children, reducing IMR and MMR, rising enrolment ratio and reducing drop out rates, universalization of primary education, increasing coverage for immunization etc. The Prime Minister's Office is quarterly monitoring the National Plan of Action for Children 2005 on the basis of eight parameters. These are as under:

- Reduce IMR to beneath 30 per 1000 live births by 2010.
- Reduce Child Mortality Rate to beneath 31 per 1000 live births by 2010.
- To reduce Maternal Mortality Rate to beneath 100 per 100,000 live births by 2010.
- Universal equitable access and use of safe drinking water and improved access to sanitary means of excreta disposal by 2010.

- 100% rural population to have access to basic sanitation by 2012.
- To eliminate child marriages by 2010
- To eliminate disability because of poliomyelitis by 2007
- To reduce the proportion of infants infected with HIV by 20 percent by 2007 and by 50 percent by 2010, by ensuring that 80 per cent of pregnant women have access to ante natal care, and 95 per cent of men and women aged 15-24 have access to care, counselling and other HIV and prevention services.

## NATIONAL PROGRAMMES RELATED TO CHILD HEALTH AND WELFARE

Several Ministries and Departments of the Government of India are implementing several schemes and programmes for the benefit of children. Some of the Schemes and Programmes being implemented by the Ministry of Women and Child Development are as under:

### INTEGRATED CHILD DEVELOPMENT SERVICES (ICDS) SCHEME

Rajiv Gandhi National Creche Scheme for the Children of Working Mothers

The Ministry of Women and Child Development has established a new Creche Scheme w.e.f. 1.1.2006 by blending the National Creche Fund with the Scheme of Assistance to Voluntary Organizations for Creche for Working and Ailing Women's Children and also to revise the financial norms from Rs. 18,480/- to Rs. 42,384/- per crèche per annum. The Scheme provides crèche services to the children of age group of 0 to 6 year, which includes supplementary nutrition, emergency medicines and contingency.

The Scheme has been named as Rajiv Gandhi National Creche Scheme for the Children of Working Mothers. These crèches will be allocated to the Central Social Welfare Board, Indian Council for Child Welfare and Bhartiya Adim Jati Sevak Sangh in the ratio of 80:11:9. The priority will be given to uncovered districts/areas and tribal areas while extending the scheme to preserve balance regional coverage. Eligibility criteria under the Revised Scheme has also been enhanced from Rs 1800/- to Rs. 12,000/- per month per family. So far about 25605 creches have been sanctioned including 5137 creches sanctioned under erstwhile National Creche Scheme upto 20th Nov., 2006

Nutrition Component of Prime Minister Gramodya Yojana and Nutrition Programme for Adolescent Girls in 51 Districts being implemented with extra central assistance given by the Planning Commission, directly and indirectly contribute to promoting nutrition of children. A National Nutrition Mission has been set up under the chairpersonship of Hon'ble Prime Minister vide notification dated 31st July 2003 with a view to enable policy direction to concerned Departments of the Government for addressing the problem of malnutrition in a mission mode.

An Integrated Programme for Street Children is being implemented by the Ministry of Women and Child Development especially for those children who are on streets and homeless and include the rag picking and vagabond children. The Scheme targets at rendering full and wholesome development of children without homes and family ties. The children without homes and family ties and children particularly vulnerable to abuse and exploitation like children of sex workers and children of pavement dwellers are the objective group for this Programme. Financial assistance is provided to the NGOs who are eligible and working for the welfare of the street children, for Formal & Non-formal Education, Shelter Home, Vocational Training to Children, Nutrition, health care, sanitation and hygiene, safe drinking water, education and recreational facilities and protection against abuse and exploitation.

## INTEGRATED PROGRAMME FOR JUVENILE JUSTICE

The programme is being implemented by the Ministry of Social Justice and Empowerment with a view to rendering care to children in difficult circumstances and children in conflict with the law through Government institutions and through NGOs. Some unique features of the scheme areas:

- Establishment of a National Advisory Board on Juvenile Justice
- Creation of a Juvenile Justice Fund.
- Training, orientation and sensitization of Judicial, administrative police and NGOs responsible for implementation of JJ Act.
- Institutional care shall be used but only as a last measure by enlarging the range of appropriate alternatives.
- Financial assistance to bring about a qualitative improvement in the existing infrastructure.
- Expansion of non-institutional services like sponsorship, foster care, probation etc as and an alternate to institutional care.

Childline India Foundation (CIF) has been set up as a nodal organization, supported by Government of India, to monitor and ensure the qualitative development of the Childline service across the country. Childline is a toll free telephone service (1098) which anyone can call for assistance in the interest of children. It has prescribed minimum quality standards for the services to be provided by its partner organizations that are implementing Childline programmes in several cities of the country. It starts preparatory activity that precedes the initiation of Childline service in any city. CIF is also involved in awareness and advocacy in order to strengthen the efforts relating to child welfare.

The target of the Shishu Greh Scheme is to promote adoptions within the country and to ensure minimum standards in the care of abandoned/ orphaned/destitute children. Grant-in-Aid upto a ceiling of Rs.6 lakh has been provided per unit of 10 children in a Shishu Greh.

## RECENT INITIATIVES

The Commissions for Protection of the Child Rights Act 2005 The Government has recently notified the Commissions for Protection of Child Rights Act 2005 in the Gazette of India on 20th Jan., 2006 as Act No.4 of 2006. The Act envisages setting up a National Commission at the National level and the State Commissions at the State level. The proposed Commission would be set up for proper enforcement of children's rights and effective implementation of laws and programmes relating to children. The National Commission for Protection of Child Rights will be a statutory body to be set up under the Commissions for Protection of Child Rights Act. The proposed Commission will have a Chairperson and six other Members, including two women members, a Member Secretary and other supporting staff. The Chairperson would be a person of eminence in the field of child development. The members would be the experts in the field of child health, education, childcare and development, juvenile justice, children with disabilities, elimination of child labour, child psychology or sociology and laws relating to children. The officers and the staff of the Commission will be provided by the Central Government. The proposed Commission would be set up for proper enforcement of children's rights and effective implementation of laws and programmes relating to children.

The Functions of the Commissions are:

- Examine and review the safeguards provided by Constitution or any law for the protection of child rights and suggest measures for their effective implementation

- Present to the Central Government, annually reports upon the working of those safeguards.
- Examine all factors that restrain the enjoyment of rights of most vulnerable children and children in need of unique care and protection
- Study treaties and other international instruments and undertake periodical review of existing policies, programmes and other activities on child rights and make recommendation for their effective implementation in the best interest of children.
- Undertake and promote study in the field of child rights
- Spread child rights literacy amongst several sections of the society and promote awareness
- Inspect any juvenile custodial home, or any other place of residence or institution meant for children for the intention of treatment, reformation or protection and take up with these authorities for remedial action
- Inquire into complaints and take suo motu notice of matters relating to:
  - — deprivation of child's rights;
  - — non-implementation of laws for protection and development of children;
  - — non-compliance of policy decisions, guidelines or and to render relief to such children,
- Take up the issues arising out of such matters with suitable authorities;
- Such other functions as it may consider essential for the promotion of child rights.

The Powers of the Commission include the following:

- Summoning and enforcing the attendance of any person and examining him on oath;
- Requiring the discovery and production of any document;
- Receiving evidence on affidavits;
- Requisitioning any public record or copy thereof from any court or office; and
- Issuing commissions for the examination of witnesses and documents.

- Forwarding any case to a Magistrate having jurisdiction to try the same and the Magistrate to whom any such case is forwarded shall proceed to hear the complaint against the accused
- Suggesting to the concerned Government or authority the initiation of proceedings for prosecution or such other action as deem fit against the concerned person/s
- Approaching the Supreme Court or the High Court concerned for such directions, orders or writs as that Court may deem essential;
- Suggesting to the concerned Government or authority for the grant of such interim relief to the victim or the members of his family, as the Commission consider essential.

## STATE COMMISSIONS FOR PROTECTION OF CHILD RIGHTS

- The Bill also provides that State Governments may constitute State Commissions for Protection of Child Rights in their State and designate a State level and other district level children's Court in their respective State.
- The Bill has similar provisions for State Commissions in respect of their constitution, reporting, functions and powers.

With the alleviation of the status of Department of Women and Child Development to an independent Ministry headed by the Minister of State having independent charge it was essential to change the above provision to make the Minister in charge of the Ministry or Department of Women and Child Development as the Chairperson of the Selection Committee for the selection of the Chairperson of the National Commission for Protection of Child Rights. Hence, the Commissions for Protection of Child Rights (Amendment) Bill 2006 was prepared which has been passed by both the Houses of Parliament in the Winter Session. The Commission will be set up once the above Amendment Bill is assented to by the President which would enable the Ministry of Women and Child Development to select the Chairperson and Members of the Commission for its constitution.

The initiatives are being taken for constitution of the National Commission for Protection of Child Rights. The Rules for implementation of the provisions of the Act in respect for National Commission for Protection of Child Rights have been notified on 31.7.2006. Ministry of

Finance have also approved certain number of posts for the National Commission. Initiatives have been taken for appointment of Member Secretary and staff for the National Commission.

## OFFENCES AGAINST CHILDREN (PREVENTION) BILL

Child abuse involves several aspects, like, sexual exploitation, economic exploitation, domestic violence, trafficking for prostitution, corporal punishment at school, and others. Consequently, the Ministry felt a need to have a dialogue on the issue so as to ascertain the views from all quarters and to formulate a consensus in order to address the issue more sufficiently and effectively. Accordingly few consultations have been made with voluntary organizations and experts dealing with the subject. It has been decided after consultation to constitute a small group consisting of representative from Government, NGOs, legal experts and social workers which will go into all aspects of the subject and after considering all existing legal provisions and others available on the subject and formulate a draft legislation to address all issues pertaining to child abuse. After wide consultations a draft Bill for Offences against Children was prepared and circulated to the State Governments for their comments and views. After obtaining the comments of concerned Ministries and Departments a draft Cabinet Note has been referred to Law Ministry for their vetting. The proposal will be placed before the Cabinet shortly.

## CHILD BUDGETING

The key objectives of the endeavour would be to analyze budgetary provisions on social sector, to identify the magnitude of budgetary allocations made by the Centre/State Governments on schemes meant for addressing particular requirements of children, to examine the trend in child particular expenditure etc. The major agenda for the exercise of child budgeting is to review resource allocations associated with children; explore ways to increase budgetary allocations for children; assess budget utilization rates for social sector and child particular programmes, identify blockages and constraints to effective utilization; identify methods for tracking expenditure and monitoring performance to ensure that outlays translate into outcomes for children

### Proposed Integrated Programme for Child Services

According to the 2001 Census, there were 427 million children in the country. There are millions of children living in the difficult circumstances. The child protection programme in India is shared between several Ministries, which have been implementing the schemes and programmes to reach out to varied groups of vulnerable children with complex and diverse needs. The significant schemes and programmes for such children include Programme for Juvenile Justice, Integrated Programme for Street Children, Shishu Grih Scheme, Scheme for Working Children in Need of Care and Protection, General Grant-in-Aid Scheme, CHILDLINE Service, Rajiv Gandhi National crèche scheme for the children of working mothers, Pilot Project to Combat the Trafficking of women and Children for Commercial Sexual Exploitation in Destination Areas, etc. However, experiences with thc implementation of existing programmes and polices has brought out a large number of shortcomings in the system.

In view of the gaps identified and recommendations and suggestions received from several quarters it has decided to combine the existing child protection schemes under one integrated scheme titled "Integrated Child Protection Scheme". The proposed scheme targets to render for care and protection of all the children in conflict with law and children in need of care and protection. It would involve steps to strengthen families and prevent them to break-up leading children to become homeless and without care and protection. At the same time, children already outside the mainstream need to be provided support beginning from emergency outreach services to final rehabilitation with their families/society. Details of the Scheme are being worked out which is proposed to be implemented in the Eleventh Plan.

## OTHER ACTIVITIES OF CHILD WELFARE

### Cooperation with UNICEF

UNICEF projects are being implemented in India through Master Plan of Operations, which is an agreement prepared after mutual consultation and consensus within the framework of Basic Agreement signed between India and UNICEF in 1978. India is the largest Country Programme of UNICEF in the world.

The Programmes are being implemented through several Ministries and Departments dealing with children which includes Ministry of Women and Child Development, Department of Elementary Education and Literacy, Department of Family Welfare and NACO, Ministry of Social Justice & Empowerment, Ministry of Labour, Ministry of Information & Broadcasting, Ministry of The parents Affairs & Sports, and Department of Drinking Water Supply (Rajiv Gandhi National Drinking Water Mission).

The Ministry of Women Child Development is the nodal Ministry for coordinating the implementation of the Master Plan of Operations. The Ministry of Women and Child Development conducts periodic review meetings to coordinate and monitor the implementation and expenditure of the UNICEF programmes in India.

The total allocation for the last UNICEF-GOI Programme of Co-operation for the period 2003-2007 is US$ 400 million. An additional funds of US $ 100 million has also been approved by UNICEF for utilization in the present MPO period.

The present Master Plan of Operations for the period 2003-07 was signed by GOI & UNICEF on 13th January, 2003.

The MPO aims to attain the following objectives:

a. To empower families and communities with suitable knowledge and skills to improve the care and protection of children
b. To expand partnerships as a way to leverage resources for children and scale up interventions
c. To strengthen the assessment and knowledge base of best practices on children.

The programme contribute towards:

a. Reduction in infant and maternal mortality
b. Improvements in levels of child nutrition
c. Ensuring universal elementary education
d. Enhancing child protection
e. Protection of children and adolescents from HIV/AIDS.

The main activities included in different sectoral programmes are given beneath:

- Education
- Child Development and Nutrition
- Child Protection
- Reproductive and Child Health
- Child's Environment: Water, Environment and Sanitation
- HIV/AIDS
- Advocacy and Partnerships

India is annually contributing an amount of Rs. 3.80 crore to UNICEF.

## CHANGING TRENDS IN HOSPITAL CARE, PREVENTIVE, PROMOTIVE AND CURATIVE ASPECTS OF CHILD HEALTH

If we see and analyze about the quantitative examination of the dynamics of hospital performance we will notice that the degree to which hospitals are making better (or degenerating) in quality and efficiency over time. Results indicate important improvements across hospitals in reducing mortality and rising efficiency over 2001-2005, with mixed results in complication and morbidity rates. Reduced mortality is likely because of improvements in care, like improved diagnostic techniques and earlier interventions, in addition to more conscientious record "coding" and changing discharge practices. Consistent reductions in length of stay underscore the financial pressures on hospitals, perhaps combined with improved ability to stabilize, treat, and discharge patients. The characteristics of the most-improving hospitals indicate that quality improvement is immanently attainable, occurring at least as much amongst small, non-teaching institutions as amongst their larger, more prominent counterparts.

Interest in making better healthcare quality has increased considerably in recent years. We have seen this interest play out in many ways, including greater emphasis on collecting and publicly disseminating performance data. In the private sector, more than half of the country's HMOs-together rendering care for more than eighty percent of managed care plan enrolees-have established "pay-for-performance" programs for doctors and/or hospitals. Policymakers have also expressed substantial interest in finding other ways to improve care, including promoting health information technology.

In spite of these efforts, it is still unclear whether the attention paid to quality measurement and public reporting has begun to improve the care people receive and, if so, to what extent it has done so. The two reports render complementary snapshots of the healthcare system, illustrating the dynamics of quality improvement both at the macro level and "on the ground" at personal hospitals.

All in all, these findings seem like good news for the healthcare system, or at least for hospital care. However, several findings and key limitations of the data should give us pause. Particularly, critics of administrative data may worry that lumping together multiple conditions could obscure finer-grained patterns of care. In fact, the investigators did detect that the number of secondary conditions increased nearly 20 percent from 2003 to 2005 in one of the databases they examined. This change could be due in part to hospitals making better their coding of co-morbid conditions, which would have reduced risk-adjusted mortality rates even without changes in care. However, the investigators also found that raw mortality rates declined over the same time stage, recommending that coding alone can't account for the observed improvements.

Another concern is that the reduced mortality rate might reflect not improved quality of care, but rather a rising focus on palliative care for the terminally ill that prompts some hospitals to discharge patients home or to other facilities rather than letting them die in the hospital. However, there is no evidence that this practice is widespread enough to account for the rather impressive changes in mortality rates. Consequently, it seems reasonable to accept the report's findings of improved care and lower costs. Yet, the evidence is not sufficient to reveal how much quality has improved or costs have been reduced.

The changes in length of stay are especially remarkable because they extend declines going back more than two decades. Improvements in outpatient care have made it easier and even prudent to discharge patients earlier than was possible a decade ago. Even though the optimal length of stay for most conditions is unknown, the fact that the mean length of stay seems to be approximately three days for all patients and just four for the elderly makes one wonder when these trends will plateau, and whether further declines in length of stay would harm patients.

The other main finding from the case studies is that there is no one prescription for improved performance, either in terms of motivational "triggers" or particular scenarios. For some hospitals, the impetus to improve might be bad publicity from high-profile errors. For others, it might be appointing a leader dedicated to change. The paths to high performance vary widely as well. One hospital created a board-level commission on quality of care even though others focused on hiring hospitalists to assiduously render high-quality care. Yet, for every institution studied, making quality a high priority and dedicating resources to improving care seemed to be critical.

## PERFORMANCE TRENDS AMONG ACUTE CARE HOSPITALS

An analysis of three different acute care hospital databases over three-year periods between 2001 and 2005 reveals main improvements in risk-adjusted mortality and efficiency, but mixed results for complications and morbidity. Using public all-payer hospital data from 12 states, Medicare data from all states, and extensive administrative and clinical data from a group of client hospitals. When these were compared the number of hospitals that illustrated steady, important improvements in risk-adjusted measures of quality and efficiency with those showing steady, important declines, or "deterioration."

## Improved Mortality Rates

Substantial reductions in mortality rates across all databases are a consequence of a falling actual "raw" mortality rate and rising mortality risk. The falling raw rate recommends that hospitals are indeed becoming improved at saving lives through improved diagnostic techniques, early interventions, improved treatments, more effective rescue efforts, reductions in errors, and other initiatives. The trend also may be attributed in part to changing discharge practices, with more deaths occurring outside of hospitals (e.g., in hospices, long-term care facilities, or homes) or during subsequent hospitalizations. The rising risk recommends that hospital patients are sicker. Factors like the aging population, rising prevalence of chronic conditions, and the growing delivery of minor surgery on an outpatient basis reduce the proportion of low-risk inpatients and raise the proportion of more complicated and severe inpatients. It also may be true that hospitals are coding patients and conditions more conscientiously and completely, which raises the risk factor. Further investigation in this field is warranted.

## Improved Efficiency

Length of stay (LOS), although not a full measure of cost, is an indication of resource usage and used as a rough proxy for efficiency in this study. A steady, important reduction in risk-adjusted LOS over time seems primarily to reflect ongoing financial pressures on hospitals to reduce costs. This also may signify improved ability of hospitals to stabilize patients more rapidly, or a trend toward discharging patients earlier and caring for them in outpatient, home, and other non-hospital settings. The former would be consistent with more efficient care, whereas the latter would not reflect either greater or lesser hospital efficiency.

One possible negative consequence of the ongoing reduction in LOS is the release of patients before they are truly ready for discharge, and/or without sufficient follow-up home care in place-an issue that has been studied and should continue to be explored as hospital dynamics and forces change. Our study, however, casts doubt on the concept that declining length of stay in addition to improved mortality rates reflect discharge of sicker patients that results in more readmissions.

### Mixed Trends

Trends in complications and complication morbidity (or simply "morbidity" in this report, defined as severe complications) were mixed. Complication rates improved but morbidity rates deteriorated in the two public databases, and the reverse trend was seen amongst the third group. Possible reasons include differences in the measurement of observed rates and inferred risks for both complications and morbidity between the public and private databases.

### Characteristics of High Improvers

Contrary to widely held beliefs that the biggest strides in quality improvement would occur at large, teaching hospitals, our analysis found that most-improving hospitals in quality tend to be smaller than average size (even after excluding the smallest hospitals), and less likely than other hospitals to be main teaching institutions. That is, the results indicate that quality improvement is quite attainable at hospitals that are not the "usual suspects." Most-improving hospitals in efficiency, however, are more likely to be main teaching institutions.

Not surprisingly, hospitals showing the greatest jump in quality most frequently started at the very lowest end of the quality spectrum, suggesting they jumped because they had the most room to improve. Conversely, hospitals showing greatest deterioration most frequently started at the top level; they had most room to fall. In addition to a normal improvement in performance over time, there appears to be some temporal regression toward the mean.

## CHILD MORBIDITY AND MORTALITY RATES

Today, children's health reflects the introduction of new health services technologies and the dramatic improvements in social and economic conditions of the past century. The infant mortality rate (IMR), one of the most sensitive indicators of the overall health of a population, declined to 6.8 infant deaths per 1000 live births in 2001-an all-time low; the IMR was 6.9 in 2003. IMR in India is 56 per thousand live births. Age-adjusted death rates continue to decline for almost all diseases and injuries.

Improvement in child mortality rates, however, doesn't tell the whole story. Rates of morbidity and disability from some conditions-asthma, diabetes, attention-deficit disorders, and obesity-have increased in recent decades. Furthermore, indicators of healthcare utilization, like immunization coverage, show that the healthcare system may not be serving many children. The demographic and social determinants that will shape children's health in the 21st century are changing. India is increasingly ethnically diverse through immigration and population growth. Children constitute an ever-smaller proportion of the population, with small political influence and limited access to public resources. Finally, the burden of individual debt and massive government deficits is being shifted to the next generation, with uncertain implications for children's healthcare access and health status.

Identifying the epidemiologic patterns of death, disease, and disability amongst children is a necessary constituent of effective health policy for young. Children have medical requirements that are different from those of adults because children are dependent on adults, are on an upward developmental trajectory, and the epidemiologic mechanism of children's health conditions differs from that of adults. The National Research Council suggested that the definition of children's health be expanded to encompass development potential and overall well being and account for the influences of biological, physical, and social environments.

## HOSPITAL ENVIRONMENT FOR A SICK CHILD

### CHILD LIFE

Child life specialists and child life assistants work in patient care fields all through the hospital and outpatient clinics. These specialists can render preparation and distraction for medical procedures, play opportunities, medical play and support.

The child life staff strives to create an environment which is non-threatening and supportive, empowering children and families to make decisions affecting their care. These healthcare professionals ought to be available to assist patients and families work through potentially difficult experiences and leave the hospital with a better understanding of their healthcare.

### PLAY ROOMS AND ACTIVITY CENTRES

Activity/play is significant for the child. They are available to patients who are not under isolation restrictions. Only patients are allowed to play in the activity/playroom. Family and friends may stay with the patient in the activity/playroom only with adult supervision. Child life specialists or assistants ought to be available to render activities for the child. VCR movies are available for personal patient use, and can be checked out by the receptionist located near the activity/playroom.

## HEALING ENVIRONMENT

The Healing Environment Program brings the fine arts into the hospital. Patients of all ages can participate in developmentally suitable art activities, like painting, drawing, sculpting with clay and other fun are projects with the art therapist or volunteers. Fun and creative activities can assist patients deal with pain, stress and boredom. Artist, like musicians, storytellers, and actors should periodically visit the hospital so that patients and their families can be involved in the arts together. Local arts organizations render much of this programming.

## RESOURCE TEACHER

A resource teacher should render educational tutoring to children who will need to be out of school for an extended period of time because of an illness or treatment. The tutoring services are provided by a certified teacher with a master's degree in Education. The resource teacher will contract with the patient's school district. In addition, the teacher will assist families who may not qualify for tutoring services but need assistance with educational questions and transitional problems that arise due to their child's illness.

## SOCIAL WORK

Social Work staff ought to be available to all families in need of assistance with supportive counselling, financial concerns, society resources and legal issues.

## PASTORAL CARE

Believing that spirituality is a significant part of healing and wholeness, the pastoral care department is dedicated to the spiritual, emotional, and physical well-being of children and their families. Chaplains should make daily rounds on patient units and are available 24-hours a day, every day of the year. Upon request, chaplains should render prayer, scripture reading, baptism, communion, anointing with oil, or other religious rituals.

## GUEST RELATIONS

The hospital guest relations specialist ought to be located at the information desk in the lobby of Children's Hospital. The guest relations specialist can render with information regarding the hospital, clinics and patient room locations as well s information on nearby hotels, worship services, restaurants, pharmacies, local attractions and more.

## FAMILY SUPPORT CENTRE

Psychological evaluation and therapy ought to be available through the Children's Hospital Family Support Centre. Licensed psychologists and social workers should render assistance to families whose children face a variety of emotional or behavioural challenges. The staff also ought to be available to offer support to family members who need assistance.

## VOLUNTEERS

Volunteers should render a variety of services all through the hospital. There ought to be volunteers reading to patients, playing games, assisting with art activities or quietly holding or talking with a child. Volunteers should also render a "snack cart" during the day and evening for visitors who choose to purchase a snack. Each volunteer ought to be carefully selected and trained to be with children and their families. All Children's Hospital volunteers should wear a distinct uniform with name tags.

## PATIENT MEALS

The hospitality department's target ought to be to render meals and snacks to the child when he or she is hungry and willing to eat. Pantries located on the patient care units should rapidly prepare the food the child wants. The menu should comprise of items child-tested and approved for comfort, interest and flavour. The clinical dieticians should write this menu to entice the appetite even though at the same time rendering the needed nutrition to assist in healing and regaining energy. The child ought to be provided with a menu comprised of foods appropriate for his or her age.

## PARENT MEALS

The children hospitals should also make provisions and facility for the meals of parents staying with the child in hospital.

## PATIENT SAFETY

The hospital is a different environment from what the children are used to, consequently the following suggestions ought to be considered for the safety of child:

- Let the child's nurse know when he or she will be alone.
- Bedside or crib rails ought to be in the highest position at all

times when the child is in the crib or bed. Crib tops ought to be available for toddlers. Children under the age of four ought to be placed in a crib unless a waiver is signed by the parents.

- When the child is up in a wheelchair, high chair, or stroller, safety belts ought to be used. The child shouldn't be left unattended even though in a high chair.
- Toys with small parts shouldn't be left in the crib.
- There ought to be no running in the halls. Shoes or slippers ought to be worn by the child when he or she is out of bed.
- Information regarding the child shouldn't be given to anyone except parent(s) or legal guardian(s), unless authorized by them.
- Parents should inform the child's care provider of any situation that is concerning them.
- Parents should understand why their child is taking a particular medication.
- If the child's medication is different from what he or she received before, parents should ask the care provider to double check (different colour or method - liquid vs. pill).

## QUESTIONS OR CONCERNS

Children's Hospital should recognize that from time to time a patient or parent may have a concern regarding care or service received.

# IMPACT OF HOSPITALIZATION ON THE CHILD AND FAMILY

## The Impact of Hospitalization on Children

Hospitalization is stressful. It is so for adults, and more for children. Sick children, who are hospitalized, are usually taken away, frequently unexpectedly and unwillingly from their home, family, school and friends; from a comforting familiarity and play, to a new place, filled with constant activity, medical procedures [which may be invasive and painful], nurses and doctors [which may not all be empathic and pleasant], and-at times-separation from their parents. In addition to being invaded physically and emotionally, hospitalized children commonly witness their parents, who are their source of strength and safety, relinquishing their control to unknown strangers.

## The Impact of Hospitalization on Family

There is extensive evidence that the whole family may be adversely affected when a child is hospitalized, particularly when it is for a lengthy period and/or for a serious or life threatening illness. The parents of sick children need not only face their child's illness and its consequent ramifications, but also the child's emotional reactions and loneliness, and their own reactions to the situation.

## THE ROLE OF CHILD HEALTH NURSE IN CARING FOR A HOSPITALISED CHILD

- Nurses have played key roles in prevention in such fields as prenatal care, immunization programs, occupational health and safety, cardiac rehabilitation and education, and public healthcare and early intervention.
- Nurses in all settings can meet health promotion requirements of patients, whether their practice is in a hospital, clinic, patient's home, health maintenance organization, private office, or society setting.
- Health promotion is primarily accomplished through patient education, an independent function of nursing.
- Health promotion should occur through the life cycle, with topics focused on infancy, childhood, adolescence, adulthood, and older adults.
- For infancy, teach parents about the importance of prenatal care, fundamental care of infants, breast-feeding, nutrition, and infant safety.
- For childhood, stress the importance of immunizations; proper nutrition to enhance development and growth; and safety practices like use of car seats and seat belts, fire prevention, and poison proofing the home.
- Identify environmental hazards, and act to reduce or eliminate them.
- Identify behavioural characteristics of individual children that may be associated with accidental liability, and caution parents accordingly. Pay particular attention to children who show the following:
  - Characteristics that increase exposure to hazards, like excessive curiosity, inability to delay gratification, hyperactivity, and daringness.

— Characteristics that reduce the child's ability to cope with hazards, like aggressiveness, stubbornness, poor concentration, low frustration threshold, and lack of self-control.

- Render anticipatory guidance about child development as it relates to accidents. Direct preventive teaching toward the intended audience, be it individuals or groups, children or adults.
- Participate in policy setting for accident prevention with great emphasis on effective public health measures.

## PRINCIPLES OF PRE AND POST OPERATIVE CARE OF INFANTS AND CHILDREN

Rendering care to childbearing families is targeted at the ideal of having every pregnancy result in a healthy mother, baby, and family unit. The nurse today faces many evolving and challenging issues in achieving this target. Such advances as in vitro fertilization and embryo freezing have afforded people opportunities once never thought possible. A rising number of high-risk pregnancies result from such factors as drug abuse, acquired immunodeficiency syndrome, late or no prenatal care, teenage pregnancies, and pregnancies in women older than age thirty-five. Technologic advances in high-risk obstetric units, foetal monitoring, sonography, and neonatal intensive care units are now rendering the means to improve maternal health and save foetuses and infants who would not have survived years ago.

Today's childbearing families have many options. The planned birth may take place in the traditional hospital setting, a birthing centre, or at home. The primary care provider may be a doctor, a certified nurse-midwife, or a lay midwife. Birth-related choices commonly include the use of labour, delivery, and recovery rooms or labour, delivery, recovery, and postpartum rooms; several birthing positions and analgesic methods; alternative pain relief strategies like hydrotherapy; and the decision to allow children and others to be present during labour and delivery. Regionalization of obstetric services has provided childbearing families with access to the technologic advances and skilled personnel capable of managing pregnancy or neonatal complications.

Economic changes in the healthcare climate have dramatically affected the practice of nursing as cost-containment considerations have shortened the hospital length of stay. Many hospitals have adopted a practice of 12- to 24-hour discharge after delivery coordinated with home healthcare follow-up.

This combination of advancing technology, pregnancy risk factors, and changing economics challenges the nurse to be a highly skilled clinician and outstanding communicator.

- Reduce anxiety associated with the procedure.
  - Reduce the parents' anxiety by determining their understanding of the procedure and the meaning it holds for them.
  - Reexplain the procedure before it begins, and answer any questions they have. Ensure informed consent is signed.
  - Render explanations during the procedure, correct misinformation they may have, and make sure they know when the results will be available and how they may obtain the results as soon as possible.
- Reduce pain and discomfort associated with the procedure.
  - Reduce discomfort by having the mother lie comfortably on her back with her hands and a pillow under her head. Relaxation breathing may help.
  - Ensure sufficient time between infiltration of local anaesthetic and introduction of needle into the amniotic sac.
  - Start I.V. fluids in accordance with institutional policy. Administer terbutaline subcutaneously or I.V. or ritodrine I.V. per the patient's facility's policy.
- Reduce potential for traumatic injury to foetus, placenta, or maternal structures.
  - Have the woman empty her bladder if the foetus is more than 20 weeks' gestation to avoid injury to the woman's bladder. If the foetus is less than 20 weeks' gestation, the woman's full bladder will hold the uterus steady and out of the pelvis. The placenta is localized with the use of ultrasound.
  - Obtain maternal vital signs and a 20-minute foetal heart rate tracing to serve as a baseline to assess possible complications.
  - Monitor the woman during and after the procedure for signs of premature labour or bleeding.
  - Tell the woman to report signs of bleeding, unusual foetal activity or abdominal pain, cramping, or fever while at home after the procedure.

## CHILD HEALTH NURSING PROCEDURES

Safety is a significant aspect of child health and well-being. Injuries are the leading cause of death for children. Additionally, injury is an important cause of childhood morbidity. Though childhood deaths from other reasons have decreased, deaths from injuries remain constant.

### Role of the Nurse

- Identify environmental hazards, and act to reduce or eliminate them.
- Identify behavioural characteristics of individual children that may be associated with accidental liability, and caution parents accordingly. Pay particular attention to children who show the following:
  - Characteristics that increase exposure to hazards, like excessive curiosity, inability to delay gratification, hyperactivity, and daringness.
  - Characteristics that reduce the child's ability to cope with hazards, like aggressiveness, stubbornness, poor concentration, low frustration threshold, and lack of self-control.
- Render anticipatory guidance about child development as it relates to accidents. Direct preventive teaching toward the intended audience, be it individuals or groups, children or adults.
- Participate in policy setting for accident prevention with great emphasis on effective public health measures.

### Administering Medications to Children

Administration of medication is usually traumatic for children. The proper approach to administration can facilitate the process and enhance the child's understanding of the importance of taking medications.

### Significant Considerations

- The manner of approach should indicate that the nurse firmly expects the child to take the medication. This manner usually convinces the child of the necessity of the procedure.
- Establishing a positive relationship with the child will allow expression of feelings, concerns, and fantasies regarding medications.

- Explanation about medication should appeal to the child's level of understanding (i.e., through play or comparison to something familiar).
- The nurse must mask her own feelings regarding the medication.
- Always be truthful when the child asks, "Does it taste bad?" or "Will it hurt?" Respond by saying, "The medication doesn't taste good, but I will give the parents some juice as soon as the parents swallow it," or "It will hurt for just a minute."
- It is typically essential to mix distasteful medications or crushed pills with a small quantity of carbonated drink, cherry syrup, ice cream, or applesauce.
- Never threaten a child with an injection when refusing oral medication.
- Don't mix medications with large quantities of food or with any food that is taken on a regular basis (e.g., milk).
- Avoid giving medications to a child at mealtime unless specially prescribed.
- For each medication administered, the nurse should know the common use, safe dosage based on the child's weight, contraindications, adverse effects, and toxic effects.
- The child must be precisely identified before medication is given.
- When preparing I.M. injections, draw 0.2 cc of air into the syringe, in addition to the correct quantity of medication. This clears the medication from the needle on injection and prevents backflow and the depositing of medication in subcutaneous fat when the needle is withdrawn.

## Calculating the Paediatric Dosage

- The nurse is responsible for knowing the safe dosage range for the medication she administers.
- Factors determining the quantity of drug prescribed include:
  - Action of the drug, absorption, detoxification, and excretion are associated with the maturity and metabolic rate of the child.
  - Neonates and premature neonates require a reduced dosage due to:

- Deficient or absent detoxifying enzymes.
- Decreased effective renal function.
- Altered blood-brain barrier and protein-binding capacity.
  - — Dosage recommendations based on age-groups are not satisfactory because a child may be much smaller or larger than the average child in the age-group.
  - — Dosages based on child's weight are more accurate; however, these calculations have limitations.
- Be alert to a prescription that would be inappropriate for a child.

## REFERENCES

Behrman R, Vaughan W. Nelson's textbook of pediatrics, 16th edn. St. Louis: WB Saunders; 1999.

MacGregor J. Introduction to the anatomy and physiology of children. London: Routledge; 2000.

Wong D. Nursing care of infants and children, 6th edn. St. Louis: Mosby; 1999.

# 3

# The Healthy Child

The evidence on early childhood strongly suggests the need to shift child health policy from the present centre on social welfare to a socio-ecologically based approach. Here we review three governing instruments, exhortation, expenditure and regulation that have been used by government and discuss the relative effectiveness of these approaches in shifting the child health policy paradigm.

There can be no greater revelation of a society's soul than the way it treats its children. Study evidence has proved that the experiences of early childhood can have a sound lifelong impact on a child's health, wellbeing and competence. The significance of the early years of life in determining future outcomes, like crime, obesity, heart disease, mental health problems and poor school outcomes has been identified and highlighted. While there are numerous factors found to regulate rising crime rates, several researchers have identified children with evidenced behaviour disorders in early childhood, academic difficulties and non-engagement in schooling, and the quality of neighbourhood supervision and support as contributing factors to criminal behaviour.

Education, literacy and other social determinants of health can regulate the coping skills of children, which render the basis of learning, behaviour and health all through life. Poverty, whether measured in absolute or relative terms, has a negative effect on children's health. Particularly, poverty is linked with developmental delay, poor school achievement and employment futures, behaviour problems, increased incidence of chronic illness, visual and hearing defects and dental problems. Parental poverty and exposure to unhealthy environments (e.g., smoking; low levels of literacy; nutrition; emotional support) reduce a child's life chances. Researches in neurobiology, neurodevelopment and early intervention show that the time period from conception to school age is a critically significant time for brain development, setting the scene for prevention of some of the identified adverse outcomes through early identification and intervention.

Consistent with the rising evidence, many governments have identified support in early childhood as a lifelong determinant of health, well-being and competence, as a matter for policy development, initiating actions to ascertain complete child development strategies for their societies. This approach calls for a whole of government response, integrating health, welfare, education and other applicable parts of government. The evidence suggests that healthy public policy for infants, children and their parents is dependent on understanding of the socio-ecological factors supported by integrated, multidisciplinary and intersectoral policy and programs.

## PRINCIPLES OF GROWTH AND DEVELOPMENT

There is a set of principles that characterizes the pattern and process of development and growth. These principles or characteristics describe typical development as a predictable and orderly process; that is, we can predict how most children will develop and that they will develop at the same rate and at about the same time as other children. Though there are personal differences in children's personalities, activity levels, and timing of developmental milestones, like ages and stages, the principles and characteristics of development are universal patterns.

- Development proceeds from the head downward. This is called the cephalocaudle principle. This principle describes the direction of development and growth. As per this principle, the child gains control of the head first, then the arms, and then the legs. Infants develop control of the head and face movements within the first two months after birth. In the next few months, they are able to lift themselves up by using their arms. By six to twelve months of age, infants begun to gain leg control and may be able to crawl, stand, or walk. Coordination of arms always precedes coordination of legs.
- Development proceeds from the centre of the body outward. This is the principle of proximodistal development that also describes the direction of development. This means that the spinal cord develops before outer parts of the body. The child's arms develop before the hands and the hands and feet develop before the fingers and toes. Finger and toe muscles (used in fine motor dexterity) are the last to develop in physical development.

- Development depends on maturation and learning. Maturation refers to the sequential characteristic of biological development and growth. The biological changes occur in sequential order and give children new abilities. Changes in the brain and nervous system account largely for maturation. These changes in the brain and nervous system assist children to improve in thinking (cognitive) and motor (physical) skills. Besides, children must mature to a certain point before they can progress to new skills (Readiness). For instance, a four-month-old cannot use language because the infant's brain has not matured enough to allow the child to talk. By two years old, the brain has developed further and with assistance from others, the child will have the capacity to say and understand words. Besides, a child cannot write or draw until he has developed the motor control to hold a pencil or crayon. Maturational patterns are innate, that is, genetically programmed. The child's environment and the learning that occurs as a result of the child's experiences largely determine whether the child will reach optimal development. A stimulating environment and varied experiences allow a child to develop to his or her potential.
- Development proceeds from the simple (concrete) to the more complex. Children use their cognitive and language skills to reason and solve problems. For instance, learning relationships between things (how things are similar), or classification, is a significant ability in cognitive development. The cognitive process of learning how an apple and orange are alike begins with the most simplistic or concrete thought of describing the two. Seeing no relationship, a pre-school child will describe the objects as per some property of the object, like colour. Such a response would be, "An apple is red (or green) and an orange is orange." The first level of thinking about how objects are alike is to give a description or functional relationship (both concrete thoughts) between the two objects. "An apple and orange are round" and "An apple and orange are alike because the parents eat them" are typical responses of three, four and five year olds. As children develop further in cognitive skills, they are able to understand a higher and more complex relationship between objects and things; that is, that an apple and orange exist in a class called fruit. The child cognitively is then capable of classification.

- Growth and development is a continuous process. As a child develops, he or she adds to the skills already acquired and the new skills become the basis for further accomplishment and mastery of skills. Most children follow a similar pattern. Besides, one stage of development lays the basis for the next stage of development. For instance, in motor development, there is a predictable sequence of developments that occur before walking. The infant lifts and turns the head before he or she can turn over. Infants can move their limbs (arms and legs) before grasping an object. Mastery of climbing stairs involves increasing skills from holding on to walking alone. By the age of four, most children can walk up and down stairs with alternating feet. As in maturation, in order for children to write or draw, they must have developed the manual (hand) control to hold a pencil and crayon.
- Growth and development proceed from the general to specific. In motor development, the infant will be able to grasp an object with the whole hand before using only the thumb and forefinger. The infant's first motor movements are very generalized, undirected, and reflexive, waving arms or kicking before being able to reach or creep toward an object. Growth occurs from large muscle movements to more refined (smaller) muscle movements.
- There are individual rates of growth and development. Each child is different and the rates at which individual children grow is different. Though the patterns and sequences for growth and development are usually the same for all children, the rates at which individual children reach developmental stages will be different. Understanding this fact of personal differences in rates of development should cause us to be careful about using and relying on age and stage characteristics to describe or label children. There is a range of ages for any developmental task to take place. This dismisses the idea of the "average child". Some children will walk at ten months while others walk a few months older at eighteen months of age. Some children are more active while others are more passive. This does not mean that the passive child will be less intelligent as an adult. There is no validity to comparing one child's progress with or against another child. Rates of development also are not uniform within an individual child. For instance, a child's

intellectual development may progress faster than his emotional or social development.

An understanding of the principles of development assists us to plan suitable activities and stimulating and enriching experiences for children, and provides a basis for understanding how to encourage and support young children's learning.

## FACTORS AFFECTING GROWTH AND DEVELOPMENT

Child development refers to the biological and psychological changes that occur in human beings between birth and the end of adolescence, as the personal progresses from dependency to rising autonomy. Because these developmental changes may be strongly regulated by genetic factors and events during prenatal life, genetics and prenatal development are usually included as part of the study of child development. Related terms include "developmental psychology", referring to development all through the lifespan and "paediatrics", the branch of medicine relating to the care of children. Developmental change may occur as a result of genetically-controlled processes known as maturation, or as a result of environmental factors and learning, but most commonly involves an interaction between the two.

Age-related development terms are: newborn (ages 0-one month); infant (ages one month - one year); toddler (ages one-3 years); preschooler (ages 4-6 years); school-aged child (ages 6-13 years); adolescent (ages 13-18). However, organizations such as Zero to Three and the World Association for Infant Mental Health use the term infant as a broad category, including children from birth to age 3, a logical decision considering that the Latin derivation of the word infant refers to those who have no speech, The optimal development of children is believed to be vital to society and so it is significant to understand the social, cognitive, emotional, and educational development of children. Increased study and interest in this field has resulted in new theories and strategies, with particular regard to practice that promotes development within the school system. In addition there are also some theories that seek to describe a sequence of states that comprise child development.

If the child development and growth is not satisfactory, it may be considered that the child is perhaps having developmental delay as a result of some genetic or environmental condition. For instance, many would assert that the child usually starts toddling between the ages of 9 and 15 months, and if it doesn't happen even after the first 15 months, the child is perhaps having some developmental problems. There are many factors, that can affect the child development and growth, and it is highly significant to keep these in mind at all times.

## EATING HABITS

Food plays quite a significant role in the child life, as it provides him with the essential materials, vitamins to bc able to grow, physically and mentally as well. Child frequently gets picky, they sometimes refuse to eat, if they don't eat sufficient or eat too much unhealthy or junk food, the child development and growth will not be satisfactory. There is no particular toddler food; they can eat a lot of things, mostly simply prepared food, with only small seasoning.

Remember also, that a child only eats ½ or even ¼ of what adults eat and thus don't make him eat more, in most of the cases he will eat as much as he likes and an amount that is enough for him, if he is not forced to eat more or is made to eat faster for instance. Rendering the appropriate food in a pleasant environment, with the family sitting down to dinner will assist the child establish good eating habits, to support his development and growth.

## SLEEP

Sleep can affect the child development and growth quite significantly as well. If he doesn't sleep enough, he will not have sufficient energy during the day, will get tired and aggressive and this will have a bad effect on his mental and physical development as well. Children need lots of sleep, in the form of daytime naps and sleeps during the night, to assure their healthy development and growth.

## PLAY

Play has a significant role in the child's life in many ways. Play will assist him develop his mental skills, his imagination and creativity. He will be able to understand the world around him more if he can play and process the things that happen to him in the world, during this play. Play will also teach him how to interact socially with other children.

And if the play involves physical activity, jumping, or running, it will also develop his physical skills. Thus, play could be considered as the necessary part of a child's life, which contributes significantly to the child development and growth.

## GROWTH AND DEVELOPMENT FROM BIRTH TO ADOLESCENCE

The longitudinal growth of an individual child is a dynamic statement of the normal health of that child. Measurements ought to be performed frequently and precisely to detect alterations from physiologic growth. Though any single point on the growth chart is not very informative, when several growth points are plotted over time, it should become evident whether that personnel's growth is average, a variant of the norm, or pathologic. Somatic growth and maturation are regulated by several factors that act independently or in concert to modify a person's genetic growth potential. Linear growth within the first 2 year of life in general decelerates but then remains comparatively constant all through childhood till the onset of the pubertal growth spurt. Due to the wide variation amongst individuals in the timing of the pubertal growth spurt, there is a wide range of physiologic variations in usual growth. Nutritional status and heavy exercise training are only 2 of the main influences on the linear growth of children. Nutritional deficits result from self-induced restriction of energy intake. That single factor, added to the marked energy expenditure of training and competition for some sports, and in concert with the self-selection of certain body types, makes it difficult to identify the personal factors responsible for the slow linear growth of some adolescent athletes, for instance, those who partake in gymnastics, dance, or wrestling.

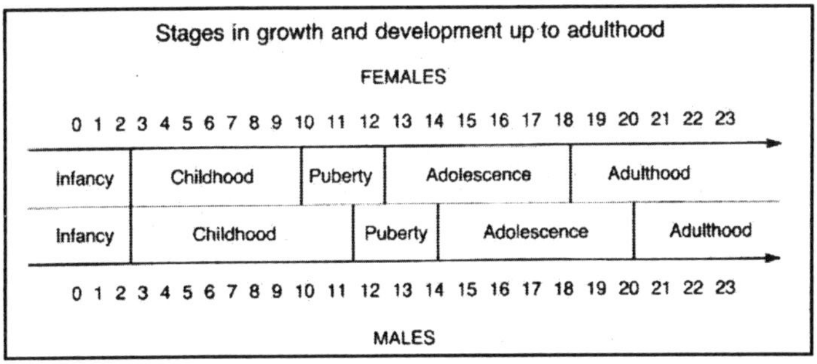


*Fig. Growth and Development from Birth to Adolescence*

A child's growth can be compared with that of his or her peers by referring to the norm on a suitable growth chart. More significant, the longitudinal measurements of a child's growth are a dynamic statement of his or her normal condition or health. Tanner has proposed that children be measured precisely to identify individuals or groups of individuals within a society who require unique care, to identify illnesses that regulate growth, or to determine an ill child's response to therapy. The linear growth of a child-adolescent athlete may also reflect the adequacy of energy intake for a particular training regimen. Measurement of growth may also be used as an indicator of the normal health and nutrition of a population or subpopulation of children.

By definition, normal (physiologic) growth encompasses the 95% CI for a particular population. Most children and adolescents who have a normal growth pattern but who remain beneath the lower 2.5 percentile (approximately -2.0 SD) are otherwise normal. The farther a person's growth falls beneath the -2.0 SD mark, the more likely he or she is to have a condition that is keeping him or her from reaching the genetically determined height potential. Cross-sectional data are derived from the measurements of many children at various ages and are in general used to derive standard growth charts. However, individual children don't necessarily grow as per these standard curves. Longitudinal growth charts derived from growth points of the same child over time more precisely describe the growth pattern of a person. In adolescence, there may be quite large deviations from the derived percentile lines, depending upon the timing and tempo of the pubertal growth spurt. An average pubertal growth pattern is built into the percentiles derived from cross-sectional data, but virtually no one person adheres strictly to that pattern.

## GROWTH MEASUREMENTS

The growth of children ought to be measured periodically and precisely. Two common devices are sufficient for such measurements and were described by Rogol and Lawton.

Neonates and infant: Small inaccuracies in length measurement can easily affect a child's percentiles on growth curve charts. Infants ought to be placed with the top of the head against the fixed headboard of the measurement device and with the eye-ear plane perpendicular to the base of the device. The child's knees must be flat against the table and the footboard moved till the soles of the feet are against it, with the toes pointing up.

Children and adolescents: Growth in children older than two years is measured with the child standing. A diurnal variation of <0.7 cm in height may occur in these children, whose height is greatest upon arising. Children ought to be measured without shoes while standing against the vertical plane to which the measuring tape is attached. The child's heels, buttocks, shoulders, and back of the head ought to be touching the wall.

The eye-ear plane ought to be perpendicular to the wall and the feet, including the heels, ought to be flat on the floor. With the child in this position, the right-angle device is lowered until it touches the top of the head, and the height is recorded on the suitable physical growth curve.

A significant parameter of growth is height velocity, which can be derived from measurements taken every 3-4 mo in infants and every 6 months in older children. Because children frequently have growth spurts, yearly growth velocities are usually more precisely determined by taking yearly measurements instead of by "annualizing" the growth velocity from time interval shorter than one year.

Growth velocity in children has a wide general range, as per the percentile along which a child is growing. Children growing along the third percentile average 5.1 cm of growth per year, whereas those growing along the 97th percentile average 6.4 cm/year for boys and 7.1 cm/year for girls during childhood to maintain growth along one of the percentiles on the growth curve. To maintain growth along the 10th percentile for height, a child must grow at the 40th percentile for velocity, whereas to maintain growth along the 90th percentile for height, a velocity at the 60th percentile is required. This implies that a child who persistently grows at the 10th percentile for velocity will progressively cross percentiles downward on the standard height curve. Some children have a small increase in growth velocity at approximately 6-7 year (midgrowth spurt), but this is not a consistent finding, and the gain in height is in general of small magnitude. Seasonal variations in growth have been noted in some children. Linear growth tends to be greater in the spring than in the fall, but weight gain is greater in the fall months. These trends emphasize the need for repeated measurements during a year to precisely assess a child's growth pattern.

Growth evaluation: Linear growth and physical maturation are dynamic processes encompassing molecular, cellular, somatic, and organismal changes. Traditionally, stature has been primarily used for growth evaluation, but changes in body proportion and composition are also necessary elements of growth, particularly of maturation. Growth standards have been derived for several populations and parameters within a population and are frequently codified into a series of growth charts. The following discussion emphasizes the genetic, nutritional, hormonal, and physical activity factors that might alter the growth process.

Physiologic Growth Patterns: Though any single point on a growth chart is not very informative, when several growth points are plotted over time, it becomes evident whether an person's growth is average, a variant of the norm, or pathologic (growth failure). The point at which a person is placed at any given time can be associated with the height age, or the age at which that child's height would be at the fiftieth percentile.

This point indicates the mean age of children of that measured height in the general population. The height age is determined from the growth chart by drawing a line parallel to the chronologic age axis from the child's plotted point to the fiftieth percentile and then a perpendicular line to the horizontal axis. The intersection of the latter line with the age axis is the height age.

Growth in several dimensions shows an important family resemblance. Adult stature, tempo of growth, timing and rate of sexual development, skeletal maturation, and dental development are all significantly influenced by genetic factors and estimates of genetic transmissibility range from forty-one% to seventy-one%. Adult stature is best correlated with calculations of midparental height (the difference in the mean adult heights of the parents), but the polygenic mode of inheritance of height leads in greater variation in the size of children born to parents of disparate heights than in children of parents who are both of medium height. Mature height can be predicted on the basis of midparental height.

The adjusted midparental height (target height) is calculated by adding thirteen cm (the difference between the fiftieth percentiles for adult men and women) to the mother's height (for boys) or subtracting thirteen cm from the father's height (for girls) and then taking the mean of the height of the same-sex parent and the adjusted height of the opposite-sex parent. Adding 8.5 cm above and beneath the midparent target height will approximate the target height range of the 3rd to 97th percentile for the anticipated adult height for that child adjusted for his or her midparental stature (genetic potential). Other methods also exist for predicting the adult stature of a person on the basis of mathematical formulations derived from the growth history of that child or from the achieved height and bone age of the child as calculated from particular tables.

The overall contribution of heredity to adult size and shape varies with environmental circumstances, and they continuously interact all through the total growth period. Children with similar genotypes, who would reach the same adult height under optimal conditions, may be differentially affected by adverse circumstances. Thus, the interaction between genetic makeup and the environment is complex and nonadditive.

The genetic control of the tempo of growth appears to be independent of that for body size and shape, and environmentally induced changes in tempo don't seem to significantly alter adult height or shape.

Somatic growth and maturation are regulated by several factors that act independently or in concert to modify a person's genetic potential. For instance, at birth, an infant's size is more dependent on maternal nutrition and intrauterine and placental factors than on genetic makeup. The correlation coefficient for adult height is only 0.25 at birth but is 0.80 by 2 year of age. There is also evidence that not all genes are dynamically expressed at the time of birth, which probably accounts for the observation that the correlation between the sizes of the parents and the child is weak during the first year of life but increases to the adult value of 0.5 by 18 mo of age.

Differences in development and growth also vary as a function of sex and ethnic origin. Sex-specific patterns in the tempo of growth, the timing of the adolescent growth spurt, overall size, and the age of skeletal maturity are well known, but differences between the sexes are evident from the time of foetal life. At birth, the skeletal maturation of females is 4-6 week more advanced than that of males, and this trend continues all through childhood and adolescence. Growth velocity is slightly slower in females at birth, becomes equal at 7 months of age, and is then to some extent faster till age 4 years.

Thereafter, children of both sexes grow at approximately the same rate till the adolescent growth spurt. On average, females enter puberty 2 years earlier than males but have a lesser peak height velocity (9 cm compared with 10.3 cm) and adult stature. Overall size and rate of development vary significantly amongst ethnic populations. Black infants tend to be smaller at birth but experience an acceleration of linear growth that results in greater height than in white children during the first few years of life. Skeletal maturity in black children, particularly girls, also tends to be more advanced and the age at peak height velocity earlier. Black girls also tend to be taller and heavier than white girls during puberty and have a tendency toward greater body mass index and greater skinfold-thickness measurements.

Growth in the first 2 years of life: Growth during the first 2 years of life is characterized by a gradual deceleration in both linear growth velocity and rate of weight gain, both of which level off at 2-3 years of age. It is during this stage that infants exhibit the pattern of growth consistent with their genetic backgrounds. Two-thirds of all infants cross percentiles on the growth curve, either upward (catch-up growth) or downward (lag-down growth). Catch-up growth typically begins within the first 3 months and is complete by 12-18 months, whereas lag-down growth commences a little later and may not be complete till 18-24 months. With the exception of puberty, the crossing of growth percentiles at any other time is cause for concern and further assessment.

Prepubertal growth: Growth during childhood is a comparatively stable process. The infancy shifts in the growth pattern are complete and the child follows the trajectory achieved previously. Till about the age of 4 years, girls grow slightly faster than boys and both sexes then average a rate of 5-6 cm/years and 2.5 kg/years till the onset of puberty. A general rule of thumb is that a child grows 10 cm (25 inches) in the first year of life, half that [12-13 cm (5 inches)] in the second year, and then 5-6 cm (2.5 inches) each year till puberty. Assuming an average birth length of 51 cm (20 inches), an average 1-years-old is 76 cm (30 inches) long, 2 years-old is 89 cm (35 inches), a 4-years-old is 102 cm (40 inches), and 8-yeras-old is 127 cm (50 inches).

Pubertal growth: Puberty is a dynamic stage of development marked by fast changes in body size, shape, and composition, all of which are sexually dimorphic. The onset of puberty corresponds to a skeletal (biological) age of 11 years in girls and 13 years in boys. On average, girls enter and complete each stage of puberty earlier than do boys. The timing and tempo of puberty vary widely, even amongst healthy children. In determining the appropriateness of a particular growth velocity, the child's degree of biological maturation must be regarded. Skeletal or pubertal maturation may be used to determine the child's degree of biological development.

The bone age is determined as the mean of the skeletal ages of several of the small bones of the hand and wrist. Pubertal maturation status is established on the development of breasts and pubic hair in girls and of pubic hair and genitals in boys. This range of general variability is expanded to an even greater degree by alterations in energy intake and expenditure. Though moderate activity is linked with cardiovascular benefits and favourable changes in body composition, excessive physical activity during childhood and adolescence may negatively affect growth and adolescent development.

Sports that emphasize strict weight control and high energy output-for instance, scholastic wrestling, gymnastics, and dancing-are of particular concern for growth disorders, though selection criteria for certain body types make selection bias a confounding variable in evaluating the effect of training on growth and adolescent development. One must consider that some of these change are transient, at least in wrestlers. The same markers of growth and body composition that are slowed during training (in season) accelerate after the season, which permits a catch-up process to control growth and cause no permanent growth reductions.

One of the hallmarks of puberty is the adolescent growth spurt. As puberty approaches, growth velocity slows to a nadir ("preadolescent dip") before its sudden acceleration during midpuberty. The timing of the pubertal growth spurt in girls is typically at Tanner breast stage 3 and doesn't reach the magnitude of that in boys. Girls average a peak height velocity of 9 cm/years at age 12 and a total gain in height of 25 cm during the pubertal growth stage. Boys, on average, achieve a peak height velocity of 10.3 cm/years 2 years later than girls, during Tanner genital stage 4, and gain 28 cm in height. The longer duration of prepubertal growth in boys, combined with a greater peak height velocity, results in an average adult height difference of 13 cm between men and women. After a stage of decelerating height velocity, growth virtually ceases due to epiphyseal fusion, typically at a skeletal age of 15 years in girls and 17 years in boys.

Puberty is also a time of significant weight gain; 50% of adult body weight is gained during adolescence. In boys, peak weight velocity occurs at about the same time as peak height velocity and averages 9 kg/years. In girls, peak weight gain lags behind peak height velocity by 6 months and reaches 8.3 kg/years at 12.5 years of age. The rate of weight gain decelerates in a manner similar to height velocity during the later stages of pubertal development.

Marked changes in body composition, including alterations in the relative proportions of water, muscle, fat, and bone, are a hallmark of pubertal maturation and result in typical female-male differences. Under the influence of the gonadal steroid hormones and growth hormone (GH), increases in bone mineral content and muscle mass occur and the deposition of fat is maximally sexually dimorphic. The changes in the distribution of body fat (central compared with peripheral, subcutaneous compared with visceral, and upper compared with lower body) results in the typical android and gynoid patterns of fat distribution of the older adolescent and adult.

Under the influence of testosterone, boys have an important increase in growth of bone and muscle and a concurrent loss of fat in the limbs.

The maximal loss of fat and increase in muscle mass in the upper arms corresponds to the time of peak height velocity. In boys, the significant increase in lean body mass exceeds the total gain in weight due to the concomitant loss of adipose tissue.

As height velocity declines, fat accumulation resumes in both sexes but is twice as fast in girls. As adults, males have 150% of the lean body mass of the average female and twice the number of muscle cells. The increase in skeletal size and muscle mass leads to increased strength in males. Both androgens and oestrogens promote deposition of bone mineral, and >90% of peak skeletal mass is present by age 18 years in adolescents who have undergone usual pubertal development at the usual time. In girls, nearly one-third of total skeletal mineral is accumulated in the 3-4-years period promptly after the onset of puberty. Adolescents with delayed puberty or secondary amenorrhea may fail to accrue bone mineral generally and have reduced bone mineral density as adults.

During pubertal development, interactions between GH and the sex steroid hormones are striking and pervasive. Researches of adolescent boys showed that the rising concentrations of testosterone during puberty play a crucial role in augmenting spontaneous secretion of GH and production of insulin-like growth factor I (IGF-I). The ability of testosterone to stimulate pituitary GH secretion, however, appears to be transient and expressed only peripubertally; GH and IGF-I concentrations decrease significantly during late puberty and into adulthood, in spite of continued high concentrations of gonadal steroid hormones. In contrast with testosterone, oestrogen modulates GH secretory activity in a disparate manner; low doses of oestrogen stimulate IGF-I production through enhanced GH secretion, but higher doses arrest IGF-I production at the hepatic level.

## VARIATIONS OF NORMAL GROWTH

Normal variants of growth were found in 82% of children whose height decreased at the third percentile (-2 SD) but in only 50% of those whose height decreased at the first percentile (-3 SD) of the mean for age. Evaluation of skeletal maturation is perhaps the best index of biological age or maturity status, because its development spans the total stage of growth. Several methods exist for determining the former. Each uses a single radiograph of the left hand and wrist and makes comparisons with children of normal stature by using an atlas and scoring system. Because girls are more developmentally mature than boys at any given chronologic age, separate standards exist for females and males.

## Familial Short Stature

On average, children of smaller parents will eventually achieve lesser height than children of taller parents. Because bone age approximates chronologic age, these children usually grow at a suitable rate during childhood and achieve sexual maturation and pubertal growth spurt at the usual ages.

## Constitutional Delay of Growth

A constitutional growth delay is regarded to be a delay in the tempo of growth. In this case, each calendar year is not accompanied by a full year of growth and skeletal development, so the person calls for more time to complete the growth process. Most of these children will eventually have delayed adolescence in addition to delayed attainment of adult stature. Birth history and birth length are in general normal, but the growth pattern shifts downward to the lower percentiles, so that the lowest values for growth velocity are obtained at 3-5 year of age. Thereafter, this pattern is characterized by steady progression of growth. Because the bone age doesn't advance one year for each calendar year, it progressively deviates from the chronologic age. The height age is usually approximately the same as the bone age, and if true, the mature height will be well within the usual range for the suitable population. Like familial short stature, this pattern is frequently familial, and because both are comparatively common, some children will have elements of both.

## Nutrition and Growth

Worldwide, the single most common cause of growth retardation is poverty-related malnutrition. Nutritional growth retardation (also known as nutritional dwarfism) and delayed pubertal development amongst suburban upper-middle- and upper-class adolescents more frequently result from self-induced restriction of nutrient (energy) intake. In addition to effects on overall growth, malnutrition secondary to avoidance of certain foods or malabsorption can lead to serious disorders, like osteopenia, anaemia, and syndromes associated with deficiencies of vitamins, minerals, necessary fatty acids and amino acids, and trace elements. Nutritional status also has an important modulating effect on the timing of adolescent sexual development. Undernutrition is linked with later age at menarche (in addition to secondary amenorrhea), whereas a moderate degree of obesity is linked with early sexual maturation. The growth curves for length and weight may at first be indistinguishable from those of children and adolescents with constitutional delay of growth or, more rarely, from those of children with familial short stature.

The diagnostic criteria for nutritional growth failure follow those of the Wellcome Trust classification. The weight for chronologic age is low, though there may frequently be a minimal deficit in weight-for-height, as occurs in constitutional delay of growth and adolescence or even familial short stature. Though the particular behaviours needed for the diagnosis of anorexia nervosa or bulimia nervosa are absent, there is deteriorating linear growth or delay in adolescent development linked with insufficient weight gain. It appears that a preoccupation with slimness and striving for weight control, fuelled by present health beliefs, cause the retarded growth. Single growth points of underweight-for-height are not nearly as significant as longitudinal data, because individuals with constitutional thinness may have a weight that is >2 percentile lines beneath their height.

Nutritional growth retardation must be differentiated from the variations of usual growth noted above and also from some of the forms of inflammatory and other bowel diseases in which growth failure, frequently noted by deviation from a previously defined length and weight channel, may be well above the lowest percentiles. Rehabilitation of nutritional growth failure or relief of the inflammation may promote catch-up growth.

The theoretical weight, the weight deficit for that theoretical weight, and the weight-for-height deficit ought to be defined. This is because children with familial short stature and mild constitutional delay of growth and adolescence most frequently continue to gain weight. This weight gain is either along an established percentile or slightly beneath but parallel to the lowest percentile on the chart. The hallmark of nutritional growth delay is that weight progressively deviates from the previous channel, an observation that underscores the importance of gathering longitudinal data.

Children with nutritional growth retardation may have reached a new energy equilibrium phase between their genetically determined growth potential and the present energy intake, because growth deceleration is the adaptive response to suboptimal energy intake. This growth deceleration has limits; for instance, energy intake (and frequently protein) may be insufficient for such a prolonged period of time that energy malnutrition becomes apparent. Acutely, suboptimal intake because of illness or heavy exercise load may temporarily delay growth, but this will be followed rapidly by catch-up growth. This process must be correctly distinguished from other reasons of organic and nonorganic growth retardation.

The adaptive response is marked by a decrement in basal (and resting) metabolic rate and a decrease in protein synthesis, the latter being an energy-intensive process. In addition, there may be deficiencies in minerals, especially zinc and iron, and vitamins. All may lead to a decrease in physical activity, which is an attempt to decrease ongoing energy losses.

## Effects of Physical Activity and Training on Growth and Adolescent Development

Does physical activity, sport training, or both affect linear growth and pubertal maturation? The literature is replete with reports that the effects of athletic training on growth and pubertal development are salutary, deleterious, or nonexistent. However, careful appraisal of these reports frequently reveals severe methodological faults, such as lack of consideration of interindividual variation in biological maturity status and subject selection. Certain sports show advantages for the early maturer, particularly for males, and others, particularly gymnastics and dance, favour the later-developing female. Thus, there is concern about the potential effects of training on the timing and progression (tempo) of puberty "caused" by participation in training and sports. Critical analysis with the biological indicators of bone age or peak height velocity in longitudinal study designs is needed to tease out the effects of such training on pubertal development and adult height.

## Females

Delay in growth and sexual maturation is well documented amongst certain groups of elite female athletes, most notably gymnasts, dancers, and long-distance runners. The underlying mechanisms, however, are not totally clear, in part due to few longitudinal data in girls. Control of growth and age at menarche involve the complex interaction of many factors, including the physical and metabolic requirements of intensive athletic training and competition.

Investigations of growth parameters in adolescent female gymnasts consistently find these girls to be shorter and lighter and to have a significantly lower percentage of body fat than do age-matched control girls or athletes participating in less strenuous sports, like swimming. Girls participating in the latter types of sports are in general taller and mature earlier than usual. Theintz et al followed a cohort of adolescent gymnasts and swimmers over a gap of 2-3 year. Training periods averaged 22 h/wk for the gymnasts and 8 h/wk for the swimmers. The gymnasts had significantly lower growth velocities from skeletal age 11-13 year, showing a peak height velocity of only 5.48 ± 0.32 cm/year compared with 8.0 ± 0.50 cm/year for the swimmers. Over time, height SD scores decreased significantly in the gymnasts without a change in the ratio of chronologic age to bone age. Therefore, predicted heights of the gymnasts decreased with time, but those of the swimmers did not change.

Lindholm et al also observed slower growth velocities amongst a group of adolescent female gymnasts. These girls did not display the distinct growth spurt seen in the control group of inactive girls, and 27% had adult heights that were less than expected established on midparental height. Bernadot and Czerwinski studied 2 groups of female gymnasts, one aged 7-10 year and the other aged 11-14 year. Weight-for-age and height-for-age decreased from the 48th percentile in the younger group to the 20th percentile in the older gymnasts. Body fat did not differ significantly between the age groups, and at all ages the gymnasts had significantly more muscle mass for their size than did the control group.

Several investigations have compared age at menarche amongst female athletes participating in different sports with that of the normal population. Claessens et al found the median age at menarche to be 15.6 ± 2.1 year amongst a group of gymnasts and 13.2 ± 1.2 year amongst the control population. Theintz et al observed that amongst a group of gymnasts and swimmers aged 12.7 ± 1.1 year, only 7.4% of the gymnasts had experienced menarche, in contrast with 50% of the age-matched swimmers. The gymnasts in this study, however, had an important delay in skeletal age (-1.42 ± 0.99 year), but the swimmers had comparable chronologic and skeletal ages. This report emphasized the importance of the interaction between somatic growth and sexual maturation and the interpretation of physiologically versus pathologically delayed puberty. Baxter-Jones et al reported the mean ages at menarche of adolescents being intensively trained in gymnastics, swimming, and tennis to be 14.3, 13.3, and 13.2 year, respectively, with a population reference value of 13.0 year. Significant delay was again noted only amongst the group of gymnasts. The data for gymnasts are replicated to a lesser degree in dancers and runners. Sports like swimming, speed skating, and tennis appear to have minimal effects on growth or age at menarche.

Though these data suggest a relation between intense athletic training and growth and pubertal development in female gymnasts, they are not conclusive. In interpreting development and growth data of athletes, a host of other variables, including the intensity of training, must also be regarded. A person's normal state of health is critical to usual development and growth, but this is assumed in adolescents who meet the great physical requirements of long-term training. Genetic predisposition also plays a significant role; the short stature of gymnasts is frequently familial and a positive correlation has been found between menarcheal age in mothers and daughters. Historically, socioeconomic class and family size have been influential; menarche occurs earlier in the higher socioeconomic classes and in families with fewer siblings. Psychological and emotional stressors linked with years-long training, frequent competition, maintenance of low body weight, altered peer relations, and requirements of coaches may also regulate growth and pubertal timing.

Nutrition, particularly dieting behaviour, can be a main factor for disordered growth, especially in sports that emphasize strict weight control. Though the principle of a critical percentage of body fat is no longer regarded valid, the issue of energy balance is important to development and growth. Intake of energy, in addition to of vital nutrients like calcium, which is essential for bone mineral accrual, may be suboptimal in athletes who restrict dietary intake during a time of increased metabolic demand. Nutter found that the desire to be thin may regulate dietary patterns of female athletes even more than do changes in exercise training.

Several investigators, for instance, Warren, have stressed the importance of strenuous physical training before menarche that might cause disordered growth and adolescent development. The younger children may be particularly susceptible to the energy requirements of strenuous exercise. Though similar trends depending upon type of sport are evident, menarche is more delayed in gymnasts than in swimmers or tennis players who started training at a comparable age. Prior menstrual irregularity appears to be a significant risk factor for oligomenorrhea or amenorrhea in adolescents who start training after menarche.

Alterations in growth and pubertal maturation are not common amongst the young women engaging in recreational exercise or in adolescents who train <15 h/wk. The incidence of oligomenorrhea or amenorrhea and secondary amenorrhea has been cited as 10-40% amongst athletes and 2-5% amongst the normal population. The distinction between elite and nonelite athletes is significant because it pertains to training time and intensity. Olympic athletes have been shown to have significantly later menarche than high school, college, and club-level athletes. The different requirements of several sports also dictate the quantity of time spent in strenuous physical activity; gymnasts and dancers far exceed swimmers and tennis players in the available researches. Catch-up growth has been reported in gymnasts when their training is temporarily reduced or stopped.

However, one of the most significant variables (perhaps the single most significant variable) to take into account is that of selection bias. Body types that are most successful are selected for particular sports. Several researches have reported gymnasts to be smaller than their peers from the young age. Delayed menarche favours the continuation of sports like gymnastics, which suggests that elite gymnasts are selected in part for this attribute. Continued participation in turn leads to more intense training and blurring of cause and effect.

The implications of delayed menarche are directly relevant to the accrual of bone mineral. Because >90% of the total adult bone mass is established during the pubertal years, failure to accrue bone mineral at a usual rate during this time may result in permanent deficits. Bone mineralization is a complex process regulated by nutrition (particularly calcium intake), weight-bearing activity, and sex steroid hormones. Hypoestrogenism due to pubertal delay or secondary amenorrhea can lead to low bone mineral density in spite of sufficient weight-bearing exercise. In a group of female runners, Louis et al found decreases in bone mineral density in all subjects with oligomenorrhea or amenorrhea, whereas runners with regular menses had values within the usual range. A low rate of bone mineral accrual has been proposed as one factor contributing to skeletal injuries in gymnasts.

## Males

Generally, boys who participate in sports have normal growth rates and are normal or advanced for their state of skeletal and sexual maturation. The advanced states of maturation in male athletes may be attributed to the power and performance advantages linked with maturation.

However, for sports that may create an energy drain, the effects on growth and maturation remain inconclusive. Seefeldt et al reported that the height velocity of elite male distance runners was equal to non-running control subjects during one year of training. Other investigations have reported the linear growth of male distance runners to be either slowed or advanced relative to reference data. Unfortunately, the maturity levels of the runners, the reference data, or both were not given for the 2 former researches, so few conclusions can be made with regard to the influence of distance running on growth velocity.

The growth of scholastic wrestlers has also been the concern of several investigations. Wrestlers start losing weight to certify for lower competitive weight classes as young as 8 year of age. In fact, several authors have speculated that the growth of peripubescent wrestlers may be slowed during the sports season. As a group, high school wrestlers are usually shorter than average for their age, though this too is probably a self-selection process for wrestling.

In a cross-sectional study, the growth patterns of 477 high school wrestlers were compared with those of a representative sample of adolescent males. The wrestler and reference groups were not different at any age for body weight, but the slope value for the gain in body weight was significantly greater for the reference sample. The reference group was significantly taller than the wrestlers after age 16.4 year, but the slope values for gain in height were not statistically different. Slope values were also compared for 13 other anthropometric variables, with few notable group differences. The investigators concluded that wrestling doesn't slow growth and maturation. However, the study did not address whether the growth rate during the sport season was slowed and, if so, whether there was catch-up growth during the non-training season.

As expected, many investigators have reported reductions in weight, fat mass, and percentage of body fat during the wrestling season. However, the fat-free mass is more conserved; most investigators report nonsignificant reductions. Still, the fat-free mass doesn't increase as one would expect for normal pubescent males. Because arm and leg strength diminish, one might suggest that statistically insignificant reductions in these variables may be biologically relevant. After the sport season, wrestlers experience accelerated incremental gains in weight, fat mass, and fat-free mass. The postseason gains in weight may be above the 99th percentile for age. Accelerated postseason gains in weight, fat mass, and fat-free mass suggest soft-tissue catch-up growth in the wrestlers. During the sport season, changes in anthropometric measures of lean tissue, like mid-arm girth and lean limb cross-sectional fields (obtained from skin fold corrected girths), also render evidence that in spite of heavy bouts of training, wrestlers can fail to accrue lean tissue during the sport season and show an accelerated accrual postseason.

A few compelling data implicate training or competition as causal in the shorter stature and decreased body mass of some pubertal athletes in particular sports. It appears likely that activities like gymnastics and dance in girls or wrestling in boys select for those participants with desirable genetic anthropometric traits. Added to this process are the interactions amongst diminished nutrition and the energy drain of training. Preliminary hormonal researches can't distinguish between constitutionally delayed puberty and a syndrome caused by sport participation. However, researches designed to make this distinction probably can't be done in adolescents. Investigations in adult women show that some amenorrheic athletes have altered pulsatile gonadotropin release, but it has not yet been possible to separate the effect of the training itself from nutritional and stress factors.

## THE NEEDS OF NORMAL CHILDREN THROUGH THE STAGES OF DEVELOPMENTAL AND PARENTAL GUIDANCE

The fundamental needs of children and changes in particular physical and mental abilities (like walking and understanding language) that mark the end of one developmental stage and the beginning of another. For stage theories, milestones indicate a stage transition. Researches of the accomplishment of many developmental tasks have established typical chronological ages linked with developmental milestones. However, there is considerable variation in the achievement of milestones, even between children with developmental trajectories within the usual range. Some milestones are more variable than others; for instance, receptive speech indicators don't show much variation amongst children with usual hearing, but expressive speech milestones can be quite variable.

A common concern in child development is developmental delay involving a delay in an age-particular ability for significant developmental milestones. Prevention of and early intervention in developmental delay are important topics in the study of child development. Developmental delays ought to be diagnosed by comparison with characteristic variability of a milestone, not with respect to average age at achievement. A case of a milestone would be eye-hand coordination, which includes a child's increasing ability to manipulate objects in a coordinated manner. Increased knowledge of age-specific milestones allows parents and others to keep track of suitable development.

## CONTINUITY AND DISCONTINUITY IN DEVELOPMENT

Though the identification of developmental milestones is of interest to researchers and to children's caregivers, many aspects of developmental change are continuous and don't display noticeable milestones of change. Continuous developmental changes, such as growth in stature, involve fairly gradual and predictable progress toward adult characteristics. When developmental change is discontinuous, however, researchers may identify not only milestones of development, but related age periods frequently called stages. A stage is a period of time, frequently linked with a known chronological age range, during which a behaviour or physical characteristic is qualitatively different from what it is at other ages. When an age period is referred to as a stage, the term implies not only this qualitative difference, but also a predictable sequence of developmental events, such that each stage is both preceded and followed by particular other periods linked with characteristic behavioural or physical qualities.

Stages of development may overlap or be linked with particular other aspects of development, like speech or movement. Even within a particular developmental field, transition into a stage may not mean that the previous stage is completely finished. For instance, in Erikson's discussion of stages of personality, this theorist suggests that a lifetime is spent in reworking issues that were originally characteristic of a childhood stage. Likewise, the theorist of cognitive development, Piaget, described situations in which children could solve one type of problem using mature thinking skills, but couldn't accomplish this for less familiar problems, a phenomenon he called horizontal decalage.

## MECHANISMS OF DEVELOPMENT

Though developmental change runs parallel with chronological age, age itself can't cause development. The fundamental mechanisms or reasons of developmental change are genetic factors and environmental factors. Genetic factors are responsible for cellular changes such as overall growth, changes in proportion of body and brain parts, and the maturation of aspects of function like vision and dietary requirements. Because genes can be "turned off" and "turned on", the person's initial genotype may change in function over time, giving rise to further developmental change. Environmental factors affecting development may include both food and disease exposure, in addition to social, emotional, and cognitive experiences. However, examination of environmental factors also shows that young human beings can survive within a fairly broad range of environmental experiences.

Instead of acting as independent mechanisms, genetic and environmental factors frequently interact to cause developmental change. Some aspects of child development are notable for their plasticity, or the extent to which the direction of development is guided by environmental factors in addition to started by genetic factors. For instance, the development of allergic reactions appears to be caused by exposure to certain environmental factors rather early in life, and protection from early exposure makes the child less likely to show later allergic reactions. When an aspect of development is strongly affected by early experience, it is said to show a high degree of plasticity; when the genetic make-up is the primary cause of development, plasticity is said to be low. Plasticity may involve guidance by endogenous factors such as hormones in addition to by exogenous factors such as infections.

One kind of environmental guidance of development has been described as experience-dependent plasticity, in which behaviour is altered as a result of learning from the environment. Plasticity of this type can occur all through the lifespan and may involve many kinds of behaviour, including some emotional reactions.

A second type of plasticity, experience-expectant plasticity, involves the strong effect of particular experiences during limited sensitive periods of development. For instance, the coordinated use of the two eyes, and the experience of a single three-dimensional image instead of the two-dimensional images produced by light in each eye, depend on experiences with vision during the second half of the first year of life. Experience-expectant plasticity works to fine-tune aspects of development that can't proceed to optimal outcomes as a result of genetic factors working alone.

In addition to the existence of plasticity in some aspects of development, genetic-environmental correlations may function in several ways to determine the mature characteristics of the person. Genetic-environmental correlations are circumstances in which genetic factors make certain experiences more likely to occur.

For instance, in passive genetic-environmental correlation, a child is likely to experience a particular environment because his or her parents' genetic make-up makes them likely to choose or create such an environment in evocative genetic-environmental correlation, the child's genetically-caused characteristics cause other people to respond in certain ways, rendering a different environment than might occur for a genetically-different child; for example, a child with Down syndrome may be treated more protectively and less challengingly than a non-Down child. Finally, an active genetic-environmental correlation is one in which the child chooses experiences that in turn have their effect; for example, a muscular, active child may choose after-school sports experiences that create increased athletic skills, but perhaps preclude music lessons. In all of these cases, it becomes difficult to know whether child characteristics were shaped by genetic factors, by experiences, or by a combination of the two.

## Research Issues and Methods

Establishing a helpful database of information about child development calls for systematic inquiry about developmental events.

Different aspects of development involve different patterns and reasons of change, so there is no simple way to summarize child development. Nevertheless, the answering of certain questions about each topic can yield comparable information about several aspects of developmental change. The following questions were proposed for this purpose by Waters and his colleagues.

- What develops? What relevant aspects of the personal change over a period of time?
- What are the rate and speed of development?
- What are the mechanisms of development - what aspects of experience and heredity cause developmental change?
- Are there usual personal differences in the relevant developmental changes?
- Are there population differences in this aspect of development (for instance, differences in the development of boys and of girls)?

Empirical research that attempts to answer these questions may follow a number of patterns. Initially, observational study in naturalistic conditions may be required to develop a narrative describing and defining an aspect of developmental change, like changes in reflex reactions in the first year.

This type of work may be followed by correlational researches, collecting information about chronological age and some type of development like vocabulary growth; correlational statistics can be used to state the connection between the two. Comparative researches examining the extent and course of development over time are the fundamental method for studying developmental change.

Such researches examine the characteristics of children at different ages. These methods may involve longitudinal researches, in which a group of children are re-examined on a number of occasions as they get older, or cross-sectional researches, in which groups of children of different ages are tested once and compared with each other, or there may be combinations of these approaches.

Some child development researches examine the effects of experience or heredity by comparing characteristics of different groups of children in a necessarily non-randomized design. Other researches can use randomized designs to compare outcomes for groups of children who receive different interventions or educational treatments.

## ASPECTS OF CHILD DEVELOPMENT

Child development is not a matter of a single topic, but progresses to some extent differently for different aspects of the person. Here are descriptions of the development of a number of physical and mental characteristics.

## PHYSICAL GROWTH

Physical growth in stature and weight occurs over the 15-20 years following birth, as the personal changes from the average weight of 7 1/2 pounds and length of 20" at full-term birth to full adult size. As stature and weight increase, the person's proportions also change, from the comparatively large head and small torso and limbs of the neonate, to the adult's comparatively small head and long torso and limbs.

### Speed and Pattern of Development

The speed of physical growth is fast in the months after birth, then slows, so birth weight is doubled in the first four months, tripled by age 12 months, but not quadrupled till 24 months. Growth then proceeds at a slow rate till shortly before puberty (between about 9 and 15 years of age), when a stage of fast growth occurs. Growth is not uniform in rate and timing across all body parts. At birth, head size is already comparatively near to that of an adult, but the lower parts of the body are much smaller than adult size. In the course of development, then, the head grows comparatively small, and torso and limbs undergo a great deal of growth.

### Mechanisms of Developmental Change

Genetic factors play a main role in determining the growth rate, and especially the changes in proportion characteristic of early human development. However, genetic factors can produce the maximum growth only if environmental conditions are sufficient. Poor nutrition and frequent injury and disease can reduce the person's adult stature, but the best environment can't cause growth to a greater stature than is determined by heredity.

### Population Differences

Population differences in growth are largely associated with adult stature. Ethnic groups that are quite tall in adulthood are also longer at birth and all through childhood, as compared to groups that have short adult stature. Males are also to some extent taller, though this is more evident in ethnic groups with strong sexual dimorphism in adulthood. Populations that are characteristically malnourished are also shorter all through life. However, there are few population differences in growth rates or patterns, except that poor environmental conditions may delay puberty and the linked growth spurt. The noticeably different age at puberty of boys and girls means that boys and girls of age 11 or 12 are at very different points in maturation and may reverse the usual sex difference in physical size.

## INDIVIDUAL DIFFERENCES

Individual differences in height and weight during childhood are considerable. Some of these differences are because of family genetic factors, others to environmental factors, but at some points in development they may be strongly regulated by individual differences in reproductive maturation.

### Motor Development

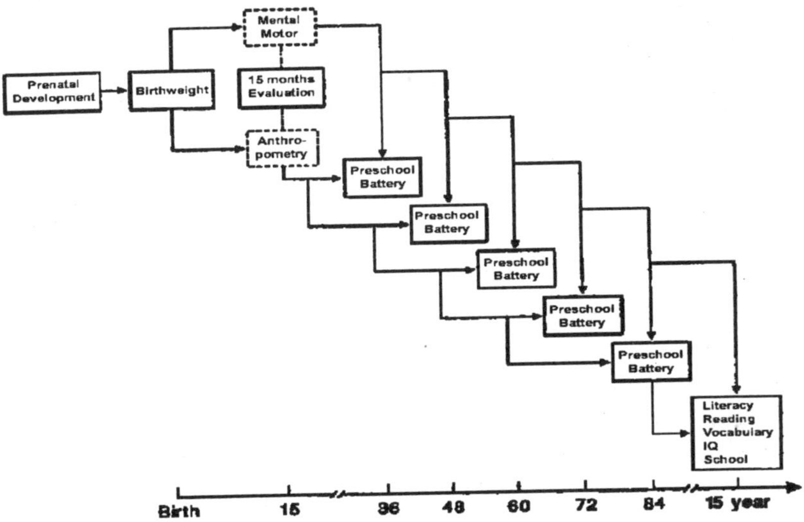


*Fig. Motor Development*

Abilities for physical movement change through childhood from the largely reflexive (unlearned, involuntary) movement patterns of the young infant to the highly skilled voluntary movements characteristic of later childhood and adolescence.

### Speed and Pattern of Development

The speed of motor development is fast in early life, as many of the reflexes of the newborn alter or disappear within the first year, and slows later. Such as physical growth, motor development shows predictable patterns of cephalocaudal (head to foot) and proximodistal (torso to extremities) development, with movements at the head end and in the more central areas coming under control before those of the lower part of the body or the hands and feet.

Types of movement develop in stage-like sequences; for instance, locomotion at 6-8 months involves creeping on all fours, then proceeds to pulling to stand, "cruising" while holding on to an object, walking while holding an adult's hand, and finally walking independently. Older children continue the sequence by walking sideways or backward, galloping, hopping, skipping with one foot and walking with the other, and finally skipping. By middle childhood and adolescence, new motor skills are acquired by instruction or observation instead of in a predictable sequence.

## Mechanisms of Motor Development

The mechanisms involved in motor development involve some genetic constituents that determine the physical size of body parts at a given age, in addition to aspects of muscle and bone strength. Nutrition and exercise also determine strength and consequently the ease and accuracy with which a body part can be moved. Opportunities to carry out movements help establish the abilities to flex (move toward the trunk) and extend body parts, both capacities being required for good motor ability. Skilled voluntary movements develop as a result of practice and learning.

## Individual Differences

Normal individual differences in motor ability are common and depend in part on the child's weight and build. However, after the infant stage, normal individual differences are strongly affected by opportunities to practice, observe, and be instructed on particular movements. Atypical motor development may be an indication of developmental delays or problems like autism or cerebral palsy.

## Population Differences

There are some population differences in motor development, with girls showing some advantages in small muscle use, including articulation of sounds with lips and tongue. Ethnic differences in reflex movements of newborn infants have been reported, suggesting that some biological factor is at work. Cultural differences may encourage learning of motor skills such as using the left hand only for sanitary purposes and the right hand for all other uses, producing a population difference. Cultural factors are also seen at work in practiced voluntary movements like the use of the foot to dribble a soccer ball or the hand to dribble a basketball.

## COGNITIVE DEVELOPMENT

The capacity to learn, remember, and symbolize information, and to solve problems, exists at a simple level in young infants, who can perform cognitive tasks like discriminating animate and inanimate beings or recognizing small numbers of objects. During childhood, learning and information-processing increase in speed, memory becomes increasingly longer, and symbol use and the capacity for abstraction develop till a near-adult level is reached by adolescence.

### Speed and Pattern of Development

It has been proposed by theorists like Piaget that cognitive development proceeds in a stage-like fashion, with qualitative in addition to quantitative differences between one age stage and others. Cognitive ability appears to move forward rapidly at times when certain achievements are apparent; for instance, the preschooler's new ability to conserve number (to know that the number of objects present stays the same although the objects are differently distributed) is an essential foundation for arithmetic and enables a number of advances. However, it is not clear to what extent evident stages are simply the results of increased speed of information processing or increased knowledge base.

### Mechanisms of Cognitive Development

Cognitive development has genetic and other biological mechanisms, as is seen in the many genetic reasons of mental retardation. However, though it is assumed that brain functions cause cognitive events, it has not been possible to measure particular brain changes and show that they cause cognitive change. Developmental advances in cognition are also associated with experience and learning, and this is especially the case for higher-level abilities such as abstraction, which depend to a considerable extent on formal education.

### Individual Differences

There are general individual differences in the ages at which particular cognitive abilities are attained, but schooling for children in industrialized countries is established on the assumption that these differences are not large. Atypical delays in cognitive development are problematic for children in cultures that demand advanced cognitive skills for work and for independent living.

### Population Differences

There are few population differences in cognitive development. Boys and girls show some differences in their skills and preferences, but there is a great deal of overlap between the groups. Differences in cognitive achievement of different ethnic groups appear to result from cultural or other environmental factors.

## SOCIAL-EMOTIONAL DEVELOPMENT

Newborn infants don't seem to experience fear or have preferences for contact with any particular people. By about 8-10 months, they go through a fairly fast change and become fearful of perceived threats; they also started to prefer familiar people and show anxiety and distress when separated from them or approached by strangers. The capacity for empathy and the understanding of social rules started in the pre-school stage and continue to develop into adulthood. Middle childhood is characterized by friendships with age-mates, and adolescence by emotions connected with sexuality and the beginnings of romantic love. Anger seems most intense during the toddler and early pre-school stage and during adolescence.

### Speed and Pattern of Development

Some aspects of social-emotional development, such as empathy, develop a case, but others, such as fearfulness, seem to involve a rather sudden reorganization of the child's experience of emotion. Sexual and romantic emotions develop in connection with physical maturation.

### Mechanisms of Social and Emotional Development

Genetic factors appear to influence some social-emotional developments that occur at predictable ages, like fearfulness and attachment to familiar people. Experience plays a role in determining which people are familiar, which social rules are obeyed, and how anger is expressed.

### Individual Differences

Individual differences in the sequence of social-emotional development are unusual, but the intensity or expressiveness of emotions can vary greatly from one usual child to another. Individual tendencies to several types of reactivity are probably constitutional, and they are referred to as temperamental differences. Atypical development of social-emotional characteristics may be mildly unusual, or may be so extreme as to indicate mental illness. Temperamental traits are thought to be stable and enduring all through the life span. Children who are active and angry as infants can be expected to be active and angry as older children, adolescents and adults.

## Population Differences

Population differences may occur in older children, if, for instance they have learned that it is suitable for boys to express emotion or behave differently than girls, or if customs learned by children of one ethnic group are different from those learned in another. Social and emotional differences between boys and girls of a given age may also be linked with differences in the timing of puberty characteristic of the two sexes.

## LANGUAGE

There are four major fields in which the child must achieve competence, regardless of the language or dialect spoken. These are referred to as phonology or sounds, semantics or the encoded meanings, syntax or the way in which words are combined and pragmatics or knowledge of how language is used in different contexts.

## Speed and Pattern of Development

Receptive language, the understanding of others' speech, appears to have a gradual course of development beginning at about 6 months. However, expressive language, the production of words, moves rapidly after its beginning at about a year of age, with a "vocabulary explosion" of fast word acquisition occurring in the middle of the second year. Grammatical rules and word combinations appear at about age two. Mastery of vocabulary and grammar continue bit by bit through the pre-school and school years. Adolescents still have smaller vocabularies than adults and experience more difficulty with constructions such as the passive voice.

Babies from one month old can produce "ooh" sounds which appear to grow out of pleasurable interactions with caregivers in a mutual "dialogue". As per Stern, this process is communication of affect between adult and infant in a mutual, rhythmic interaction. The attunement and "gaze-coupling" in which infant and adult take different roles is thought to anticipate the give-and-take of later dialogue.

From about 6 to 9 months babies produce more vowels, some consonants and "echolalia", or the frequent repetition of sounds such as "dadadada" which appear to have some phonetic characteristics of later speech. It is thought that a vital part of the development of speech is the time carers spend "guessing" what their infants are trying to communicate thus integrating the child into their social world. The attribution of intentionality to the infant's utterances has been called "shared memory" and forms a complex series of actions, intentions and actions in response in an improvised way.

It has been argued that children's phonological systems develop in ways that are parallel to adult languages, even if they are using unrecognisable "words". First words have the function of naming or labelling but also condense meaning as in "milk" meaning "I want milk". Vocabulary typically grows from about 20 words at 18 months to around 200 words at 21 months. From around 18 months the child starts to combine words into two word sentences. Typically the adult expands it to clarify meaning. By 24-27 months the child is producing three or four word sentences using a logical, if not strictly correct, syntax. The theory is that children apply a fundamental set of rules like adding 's' for plurals or inventing simpler words out of words too complicated to repeat such as "choskit" for chocolate biscuit. Following this there is a fast appearance of grammatical rules and ordering of sentences. There is frequently an interest in rhyme, and imaginative play often includes conversations. Children's recorded monologues give insight into the development of the process of organising information into meaningful units.

By three years the child is beginning to use complex sentences, including relative clauses, though still perfecting several linguistic systems. By five years of age the child's use of language is very similar to that of an adult. From the age of about three children can indicate fantasy or make-believe linguistically, produce coherent individual stories and fictional narrative with beginnings and endings. It is argued that children devise narrative as a way of understanding their own experience and as a medium for communicating their meaning to others. The ability to engage in extended discourse emerges over time from regular conversation with adults and peers. For this the child needs to learn to combine his perspective with that of others and with outside events and learn to use linguistic indicators to show he is doing this. They also learn to adapt their language depending upon to whom they are speaking. Typically by the age of about 9 a child can recount other narratives in addition to their own experiences, from the perspectives of the author, the characters in the story and their own views.

## Mechanisms of Language Development

Though the role of adult discourse is significant in facilitating the child's learning, there is considerable disagreement amongst theorists about the extent to which children's early meanings and expressive words arises directly from adult input as opposed to intrinsic factors relating to the child's cognitive functions. Findings about the initial mapping of new words, the ability to decontextualise words and refine meaning are diverse. One hypothesis is known as the syntactic bootstrapping hypothesis, referring to the child's ability to infer meaning from cues, using grammatical information from the structure of sentences.

Other is the multi-route model in which it is argued that context-bound words and referential words follow different routes; the first being mapped onto event representations and the latter onto mental representations. In this model, though parental input has a critical role, children rely on cognitive processing to establish subsequent use of words. However, naturalistic study on language development has indicated that preschoolers' vocabularies are strongly linked with the number of words addressed to them by adults.

There is as yet no single accepted theory of language acquisition. Present explanations vary in emphasis from learning theory, with its emphasis on reinforcement and imitation (Skinner), to biological, nativist theories, with innate underlying mechanisms (Chomsky and Pinker), to a more interactive approach within a social context (Piaget and Tomasello). Behaviourists argue that given the universal presence of a physical environment and, usually, a social environment, any theory of language must account for the effects of the contingent relations of these on an individual's development of language behaviour. Pinker argues that complex language is universal and has an innate basis. Pinker's argument is partly established on the development of Creole languages from pidgins.

The children of parents, who communicate, without grammatical structures, in pidgin, develop a Creole language of their own accord, complete with standardised word orders, markers for present, future and past tenses and subordinate clauses. There is some support for this from the development of sign language amongst deaf children thrown together at a young age in special schools in Nicaragua who spontaneously developed a pidgin which was then developed into a Creole by a younger generation of children coming into the schools.

## Individual Differences

Slow Expressive Language Development (SELD) a delay in the use of words coupled with general understanding, is characteristic of a small proportion of children who later display usual language use.

Dyslexia is an important topic in child development as it affects approximately 5% of the population (in the western world). Essentially it is a disorder whereby children fail to achieve the language skills of reading, writing and spelling commensurate with their intellectual abilities. Dyslexic children show a range of differences in their language development, from subtle speech impairments to mispronunciations to word-finding difficulties.

The most common phonological difficulties are limitations of verbal short-term memory and phonological awareness. Such children frequently have difficulties with long-term verbal learning like months of the year, learning tables, left and right or a foreign language. From the late 1980s the phonological deficit hypothesis has become the dominant explanation. The difficulties in early articulation, fundamental phonological skills and acquiring fundamental building blocks means that dyslexics have to invest too many resources in just coping with the basics instead of acquiring new information or skills. Early identification enables children to receive assistance before they fail.

Atypically delayed language development may be diagnostic of autism, and regression of language may indicate serious disabilities such as Rett syndrome. Poor language development also accompanies normal developmental delays like those found in Down syndrome.

## NUTRITIONAL NEEDS OF CHILDREN & INFANTS

Babies' nutritional needs are met completely through mother's milk or iron-fortified infant formula till they are about six months old. World Health Organization suggests that all infants be exclusively breastfed for the first six months of life. Mother's milk is the perfect nutrition and is quite enough to support development and growth during this time. The healthcare provider may suggest a Vitamin D supplement for the exclusively breastfed infant. Around the age of four to six months, babies start to observe and mimic their parents' or other caregivers' eating habits. At this point, the baby may be ready to graduate to "complementary" foods. Naturally, parents, grandparents and other care providers have many questions about this significant milestone: When are babies ready for solid foods? Which foods ought to be given? How much food is sufficient? This brochure provides general guidelines for introducing infants to solid foods, in addition to tips for keeping mealtime safe. Keep in mind that each baby is a person and may be ready for different foods established on age, nutritional needs, development and other factors. Ask the paediatric nurse practitioner, paediatrician, family doctor, or other healthcare provider for particular feeding advice.

**7 to 9 Months**

- Babies are ready to increase the variety of foods, in addition to the textures of foods in their diet.
- Meats, poultry, and soft, chunky baby foods may be introduced at this time.
- Breastfed babies may desire fewer feedings and formula fed babies may take less than 28 ounces of formula per day.
- Home-prepared foods ought to be steamed, and then mashed. Don't use honey or corn syrup, as they may contain botulism spores, which can be unsafe to infants. The baby will enjoy spices and herbs in their food, but shouldn't have salt or sugar added to foods.
- At this time, many babies are ready to start finger foods. The baby ought to be able to sit up straight, be able to grasp food with his or her hands or finger tips, and move the food from the hand to the mouth.
- Finger foods like chopped pieces of ripe banana, dry unsweetened cereal, crackers, or teething biscuits are good choices.

**10 to 12 Months**

- Chopped table food, well-cooked vegetables (without salt or sugar), cottage cheese and other soft or lumpy foods may be introduced.
- Babies use their gums and tongue to mash the lumps, so it does not matter if the baby has no teeth.
- Most babies eat three or four meals a day.
- Bit by bit, babies grow more independent and can be encouraged to hold a spoon when being fed and to use both hands while drinking from a cup.
- Talk to the baby by naming the food being eaten, objects in the field, the utensils used, or the colour of the food. Remember: make each feeding a special time for the parents and the baby to communicate.

If the family has a history of food allergies, it is best to breastfeed for as long as possible and to delay the introduction of solid foods till six months of age. It may be useful to delay the introduction of those particular foods that have caused allergic reactions in the family — in addition to certain foods like wheat, egg white, soybeans, citrus, peanuts, tree nuts or cows' milk, which are common sources of food allergies - till well after the first year of life. Ask the healthcare provider for particular dietary advice. By about one year of age, most babies eat small, tender table foods or toddler foods. Breastfeeding continues as long as baby and mother desire. Whole cow's milk can be introduced in the range of 16-24 ounces per day.

Children need the fat in mother's milk or whole cow's milk for proper development and growth. Consequently, low-fat milk shouldn't be introduced till two years of age. In the second year, consider introducing foods with fibre, like multi-grain cereals and 100% whole wheat bread. Avoid peanut butter till after the second year due to allergies and choking.

### 12 to 18 Months

The minimum quantity of food that children in this age range should eat includes:

- Mother's milk or whole milk 16 to 24 ounces per day.
- Fruits and vegetables 4 to 8 tablespoons.
- Breads and cereals 4 servings (a child's serving is 2 tablespoons of pasta, potatoes or rice or 1/4 slice of bread.)
- Meat, poultry or fish 2 servings per day or one tablespoon or 1/2 ounce each.

## SAFETY AT THE PLATE

When feeding children under four years of age, or children with developmental disabilities, extraordinary care is needed with foods that require extensive chewing, or could cause choking if swallowed whole. Foods like chunks of meat or cheese, hot dogs or hot dog coins, whole grapes, nuts, chunks of peanut butter, seeds, potatoes, cherry tomatoes, raw fruits or vegetables, hard or sticky candy, popcorn and raw carrots can be dangerous if swallowed whole.

Simple guidelines ought to be followed when watching children:

- Always supervise children while eating. Choking incidents frequently occur when older siblings offer babies food they're not yet developmentally ready to handle.
- Encourage children to take small bites and chew their foods completely. The young children have a tendency to bite off more than they can chew at any one time.

- Insist children sit down during mealtime or snacks. Never let them lie down while eating.
- Do not let children run with anything in their mouths.
- Cut foods into small pieces (less than 1/4 inch) and place only a few pieces on the plate at a time.
- Carefully select a sturdy high chair with safety straps.

## START OF GIVING OTHER FOODS TO CHILD

- The baby gets all the nutrients required for development and growth from mother's milk or iron-fortified infant formula for the first four to six months of life.
- The baby's risk for having an allergic reaction to food is lower when the parents wait till about four to six months of age to introduce solids, particularly if there is a family history of food allergies.
- The baby is not ready to digest foods other than mother's milk or infant formula till about four to six months of age.
- The baby will not sleep any better if solid food is added to the food before the age of about four to six months.
- The baby's risk for choking is higher before about four to six months of life because of lack of developmental readiness.

Significant recommendations about starting solids:

- The best first food is a single-grain (usually rice) iron fortified baby cereal. Rice cereal is easily digested and is not likely to cause a food allergy.
- Mix 1 - 2 teaspoons of dry cereal with sufficient mothers' milk or formula to make it such as thin gravy.
- Use a small spoon with a long handle and a rubber coating at the feeding tip to serve the cereal.
- Start feeding slowly. Place a small portion of cereal in the middle portion of the baby's tongue.
- Don't use a baby bottle to feed cereal or other solid foods to the baby. A baby needs to experience how foods taste and feel in their mouth.
- Remember that every new food is a new sensation in taste and texture for the baby. Babies may make a face and may push the food out of their mouth when a new food is introduced. It

may take 10 to 15 attempts before the baby is eager to eat a new food. This is normal. Do not be discouraged. Soon the baby will become more accustomed to eating all kinds of new foods and will eventually open his or her mouth in anticipation.

- Increase the quantity and thickness of the cereal once the baby becomes used to the consistency. Feedings will bit by bit increase to 4-6 tablespoons of cereal twice a day.
- Always make sure the baby is sitting up to eat.
- Position the baby so that he or she can see the face of the person feeding him or her. Mealtimes render significant opportunities for babies and their caregivers to smile, laugh, talk, and enjoy being together.

  Baby's appetite can vary from day to day. Babies let the parents know they are full by turning their heads away from the spoon or holding their lips closed. Never force them to eat more fod after indicating fullness. Respect the baby's appetite by paying attention to their signals of fullness. This assists the baby learn to eat just the right quantity, instead of eating too much. Knowing the signs of fullness helps avoid a problem with obesity later in childhood.

When to add other foods?

- Once the baby has mastered cereal, introduce prepared, strained baby food vegetables and fruits.
- Introduce one new food every 3-5 days to allow the child's system to adapt and to watch for any unusual reactions.
- Start with one-2 teaspoonfuls of strained or pureed vegetables, like squash, peas, carrots or sweet potatoes. These foods contain no wheat, milk, egg, or citrus to which some babies may be sensitive.
- Bit by bit increase the quantity of vegetables or fruit to about 4 to 8 tablespoons daily, depending upon the baby's appetite.
- By age seven months, the baby ought to be eating two meals of cereal, fruit and vegetables per day, in addition to continuing to breastfeed or take formula.
- Juices are not required at this age. Wait till the baby is using a cup to offer juices to protect his or her teeth from tooth decay.

## BABY FRIENDLY HOSPITAL CONCEPT

Baby-friendly hospital is a designation awarded by the World Health Organization and the United Nations Children's Fund to hospitals worldwide that foster evidence based strategies concerning infant feeding. These strategies have as an outcome an increased likelihood of informed decision making regarding infant feeding and greater skills for mothers to start and sustain breastfeeding. It is termed baby friendly because it is a global strategy inclusive of and useful to all mothers regardless of how they decide to feed their infants. The designation is awarded as per stringent criteria. The award recognizes facilities that offer mothers the information, confidence and skills required to successfully start and continue breastfeeding their babies.

The initiative was launched in 1991 as part of an effort to promote nursing over formula feeding. In developing countries, formula feeding is linked with higher infant mortality and higher social and economic costs. Even in developed countries, breastfeeding offers nutritional, developmental, immunologic, and psychological advantages.

The criteria for designation as Baby-Friendly include:

1. Have a written breastfeeding policy that is routinely communicated to all healthcare staff.
2. Train all healthcare staff in skills essential to implement this policy.
3. Inform all pregnant women about the benefits and management of breastfeeding.
4. Assist mothers start breastfeeding within one half-hour of birth.
5. Show mothers how to breastfeed and preserve lactation, even if they ought to be separated from their infants.
6. Give newborn infants no food or drink other than breast milk, not even sips of water, unless medically indicated.
7. Practice rooming in - that is, allow mothers and infants to remain together 24 hours a day.
8. Encourage breastfeeding on demand.
9. Give no artificial teats or pacifiers (also called dummies or soothers) to breastfeeding infants.
10. Foster the establishment of breastfeeding support groups and refer mothers to them on discharge from the hospital or clinic.

The program also restricts use by the hospital of free formula or other infant care aids provided by formula companies. Between 1991 and 2005, approximately 15,000 facilities worldwide have been inspected and accredited as "Baby-Friendly." The notion of "rooming in" is rapidly being converted to the notion of bedding in, where the neonate is transferred to the mother within 30 minutes after a usual vaginal delivery and maximum of 4 hours following a caesarean section.

## VALUE OF PLAY AND SELECTION OF PLAY MATERIAL

Children are being stripped of their natural creativity by structured activities and hi-tech toys, leading academics warned yesterday. Innate play skills are lost as parents pay for them to attend classes and clubs or buy televisions and video game machines for their bedrooms. Even at school they are told what games to play in sports lessons and sometimes even in the playground. But the regimentation of their leisure time is stifling their initiative, says a report.

Entitled the Trouble With 21st Century Kids, it was compiled by Peter Smith, professor of psychology at Goldsmiths College, University of London, and nutritionist Rachel Biggins. It says: "Some structuring of play can be useful now and then to get children going or assist children who have difficulty playing. But this shouldn't go too far.

Regimented play activities can have negative consequences on the social and emotional development of a child because they are too organised and take away a child's initiative and freedom of choice. In contrast, freeform play encourages the creative and multi-sensory development of a child because it has no structure."

It adds: "Play or games with rules, where it is the outcome that motivates the participation, train a child's thought patterns, leaving less time for their imagination or creative thought process to establish itself and mature." The report warns of the stifling potential of television and videos.

"Though it can be said that there are some positive effects to these activities, like hand-eye co-ordination, there is growing concern that children are spending too much time on sedentary, solitary pursuits that can arrest their mental and physical well-being," it says. "Experts agree that pre-programmed electronic toys monopolise the brain, because children respond to a scenario constructed by someone else and this is having an impact on their creativity."

Supportive adults need to home in on what kinds of play experiences and resources work best for under-threes. They also need to notice those aspects of learning-rich play that don't change across the years of early childhood: the continuing need for time, resources, space and companions.

## TIME AND TIMING

All children need enough time to enjoy their play and become deeply involved on their own terms. Adult planning has to be established on flexible timing that enables plenty of 'do it again' and 'come back to it later'. Adult-started, unique activities have to be open-ended in terms of the play experience itself and adult expectations for learning.

Toddlers and two-year-olds may use a collection of simple musical instruments to search deliberate sound-making and simple tunefulness. However, the children will be pushing the boundaries of their own learning just as much if they find a small drum will balance on its side or a circular xylophone will roll.

Practitioners can't plan and time activities with firm learning intentions that are laid down before the children have even seen the resources. None of the Birth to Three guidance tells practitioners to target for this impossible target. Instead, practitioners need to adopt a complete approach that combines giving children the freedom to make spontaneous choices about their play with unique experiences. Such an approach will encourage many aspects of a child's development, and an alert practitioner will recognise and respond to the progress made.

## PLAY RESOURCES

Children need enough resources, although many need not be bought. What is significant is that these resources are versatile enough to give children the scope to determine, influence or modify how they are used - today, tomorrow, next week. Resources used in treasure baskets and heuristic play, as pioneered by Elinor Goldschmied, point the way for a more general approach to play materials for the young children.

Goldschmied's concerns, from the late 1970s, about the limited nature of many commercial toys, are as relevant as ever. There are now even more plastic toys and items with extremely limited scope for developing children's playful interactions, imagination and learning - regardless of the manufacturers' claims.

When planning play opportunities, practitioners also need to consider how the resources will be made available. Books need to be presented on a low shelf or in a basket, a treasure trove of soft cloths in a nice basket, simple construction materials in sturdy containers. Older toddlers and two-year-olds should have easy access to imaginative play props or small world people and animals that make sense to them, as they know enough about their world to re-explore it through simple pretend play.

## SPACE AND SPACES

The young children need plenty of space, but how much ought to be determined by the resources and games on offer? They need lots of open space to spread out and move at speed: happily practicing their skills of movement and balance or playing a game of crawling-chasing with the parents. The younger, and slightly older, children need smaller, snuggling-in spaces, where they may choose to settle down with a teddy or friends to organise their own game.

Practitioners need to keep an eye on the play space available, so that there is sufficient room for an older baby or toddler to focus on their collection of soft scarves or for a two-year-old to build a brick tower and knock it down.

## PLAYFUL COMPANIONS

Sometimes babies and young children want to play on their own but enjoyable play includes the possibility of play companions - adults and other children - joining in without taking over. Practitioners need to be playful companions who sometimes follow a child's lead and sometimes introduce a new element into a familiar game.

Adult playmates can ease any tensions and role model social skills when babies and very young children want to play together but are struggling with space, turn-taking and what this game is all about today.

## AGE APPROPRIATE TOYS AND GAMES

- 0-3 months: Wind chimes, unbreakable mirrors (babies tend to look right 80% of the time so make sure the parents put any objects in their line of vision), high contrasting mobiles, cloth books.
- 3-6 months: Baby plays gyms, rattles, squeaky rubber toys, colourful teethers, and socks with bells.
- 6-9 months: Textured books, soft blocks to knock down, activity boards, toys that pop up when the baby pushes the button, balls - throw the ball and encourage the baby to crawl after it.

- 9-12 months: Walker, rocker, toy, telephone, shape sorter, books with flaps, bucket and spade for natural sand play - the baby will love the texture.
- 12-18 months: Simple puzzles like cut-out circles and squares, stacking, pull toys for confident walkers; climbing frame, washable non-toxic crayons, ride-on vehicle, toy buggy.
- 18-24 months: Musical instruments like keyboards, drum, plastic tea set, play house or den (throw a blanket on the old baby gym), shopping trolley, gardening tools, building blocks.
- 24-36 months: Illustrated books, dressing-up clothes, child-size household equipment, construction toys, e.g. Lego, wooden puzzles, dolls to undress.
- 36 months +: Basic jigsaw puzzles, memory games like snap, child-size pots and pans, plasticine, bats and balls, golf sets, reference books.

## PREVENTIVE IMMUNIZATION

Immunization is a way of protecting the human body against infectious diseases through vaccination. Immunization prepares our bodies to fight against diseases in case we come into contact with them in the future.

Babies are born with some natural immunity which they get from their mother and through breast-feeding. This gradually wears off as the baby's own immune system starts to develop. Having the child immunized gives additional protection against illnesses which can kill.

Even if the baby is brought late for vaccinations, she should still receive all the vaccinations. While it is the best to follow the perfect immunization time table, on no account should the baby be denied vaccinations, even if she is brought late for them. But every attempt must be made to complete full immunization, before the age of 1 year.

About 4 to 6 weeks after B.C.G. injection a small lump called a papule appears at place of the injection which may later break, giving out a whitish discharge. This will heal in about 10 to 12 weeks after the injection has been given and will leave a scar. Only if the discharge continues without the wound drying up, should the physician be consulted.

## SIDE EFFECTS OF VACCINATIONS

Only very few infants and children develop side effects after a vaccination. We have already discussed the side effects of the B.C.G.

After the D.P.T. injection, the infant may have pain at the site of the injection and may even develop fever. In that case the baby may be given 1/2 a table or 1/2 a tsp. of paracetamol.

After the measles injection, measles like rashes may appear. These are usual. Very rarely, children can have allergic reactions straight after immunization. Also if the baby develops high fever or loses consciousness, a physician ought to be consulted promptly. People giving immunizations are trained to deal with allergic reactions and if the child is treated rapidly, he or she will recover fully. Occasionally it is not possible to take the baby for the second and third vaccinations after precisely a month.

No, a slight delay does not matter. Continue the vaccinations according to the timetable and complete the course as soon as possible. The child will be fully protected only after she has received one B.C.G. injection. Three D.P.T. injections, 3 O.P.V. doses and one measles injection. Hence, it is very significant to take the baby for the vaccination at the correct time and to make sure that all the vaccinations are given.

There are very few reasons why a child should not be immunized. Ordinarily common illnesses such as a cold or a diarrhoea are not impediments against getting the child vaccinated.

There are certain situations although, where the parents must let the healthcare provider know of the child's conditions. Following are some of them:

- The child has a high fever;
- He has had a bad reaction to another immunization;
- He has had a severe reaction after eating eggs; or
- Has had convulsions (fits) in the past. (With the right advice, children who have had fits in the past can be immunized.)
- He has had, or is having, treatment for cancer;
- He has any illness which affects the immune system, for instance, HIV or AIDS.
- He is taking any medicine which affects the immune system, for instance, immunosuppressants (given after organ transplant or for malignant disease) or high-dose steroids.

Vaccines like all other medicines under go extensive and rigorous tests regarding their safety. Only after the have been found to be safe that they are introduced for normal vaccination programs. Each vaccine is continually checked even after it has been introduced and action is taken if it is required. If a vaccine is not safe it is not used.

**IDEAL IMMUNIZATION SCHEDULE FOR THE INFANTS**
**(Ministry of Health, Govt. of India)**

| | |
|---|---|
| **At 11/2 months** | B.C.G. (injection)*<br>D.P.T. - 1 (injection)and<br>O.P.V. - 1 (dose) |
| **At 21/2 months** | D.P.T. - 2 (injection)and<br>O.P.V. - 2 (dose) |
| **At 31/2 months** | D.P.T. - 3 (injection) and<br>O.P.V. - 3 (dose) |
| **At 9 months** | Measles (injection) |
| **16 to 24 months** | D.P.T. Booster (injection) and<br>O.P.V. Booster (dose) |

* If the infant has been delivered in a hospital/clinic, she should be given the B.C.G. injection at birth.

Preventive and Social Medicine (PSM) is comparatively a new branch of medicine. It is frequently believed to be synonymous with Community Medicine, Public Health, and Community Health in India. All these share common ground, i.e. prevention of disease and promotion of health. In short, PSM provides complete health services ranging from preventive, promotive, curative to rehabilitative services. The importance of the speciality of PSM has been very well recognised and emphasized repeatedly from grass root to international levels, not only in health sector but in other related sectors too. Whereas clinical specialities look after personal patient, PSM has to think and act in terms of whole society. The scope of medicine has expanded during the last few decades to include not only health problems of individuals, but those of communities as well. If we want to attain Health For All, Community Medicine will definitely be the key factor during the next millennium.

## GENESIS AND EVOLUTION

The industrial revolution of the eighteenth century while bringing affluence also brought new problems - slums, accumulation of refuse and human excreta, overcrowding and a variety of social problems. Frequent outbreaks of cholera added to the woes Chadwick's report on 'The Sanitary Conditions of Labouring Population (1842)' focussed the attention of the people and Government on the urgent need to improve public health. Filth and garbage were recognised as man's greatest enemies and it lead to great sanitary awakening bringing Public Health Act of 1848 in England, in acceptance of the principle that the state is responsible for the health of the people. The act was made more comprehensive in 1875 when Public Health Act 1875 was enacted.

Public Health is defined as the process of mobilising local, state, national and international resources to solve the main health problems affecting communities and to attain Health For All by 2000 AD.

While Public Health made fast strides in the western world, its progress has been slow in the developing countries like India where the major health problems continue to be those faced by the western world 100 years ago. The establishment of the World Health Organization (WHO) rendering a Health Charter for all people provided a great fillip to the public health movement in these countries.

Many different fields contributed to the growth of Public Health; doctors diagnosed diseases; sanitary engineers built water and sewerage systems; epidemiologists traced the sources of disease outbreaks and their modes of transmission; vital statisticians provided quantitative measures of births and deaths; lawyers wrote sanitary codes and regulations; public health nurses provided care and advice to the sick in their home; sanitary inspectors visited factories and markets to enforce compliance with public health ordinances; and administrators tried to organise everyone within the limits of the health departments budgets.

Public Health thus involved Economics, Sociology, Psychology, Law, Statistics, and Engineering in addition to biological and clinical sciences. Soon another significant and emerging branch of medicine i.e., Microbiology became an integral part of Public Health. Public Health during the 19th Century was around sanitary regulations and the same underwent changes.

Preventive Medicine developed as a branch of medicine distinct from Public Health. By definition, preventive medicine is applied to 'healthy' people, customarily by actions affecting large numbers or populations. Its primary target is prevention of disease and promotion of health. It got a firm foundation only after the discovery of causative agents of diseases and the establishment of the germ theory of disease. The development of laboratory methods for the early detection of disease was a further advance.

Social Medicine has varying meanings attached to it. By derivation, it is the study of man as a social being in his total environment. It may be identified with care of patients, prevention of disease, administration of medical services; indeed with almost any subject in the extensive field of health and welfare. In short, social medicine is not a new branch of medicine but rather a new orientation of medicine to the changing requirements of man and society.

Community Medicine has been defined as that speciality which deals with populations and comprises those physicians who try to measure the requirements of the population, both sick and well, who plan and administer services to meet those requirements, and those who are engaged in study and teaching in the field.

Decades old notion of healthcare approach has experienced a dramatic change. Today health is not merely an absence of disease; it is associated with quality of life instead. Health is believed to be a means of productivity. Thus, health development is necessary to socio-economic development as a whole. Because health is an integral part of development, all sectors of society have an effect on health. Scope of medicine has extended from person to society. Study of health and disease in population is replacing study of disease in man. Germ theory of disease gave place to newer notions - multi-factorial causation. Social and behavioural aspects of the disease have been accorded a new priority.

Contemporary medicine is no longer solely an art and science for the diagnosis and treatment of diseases. It is also the science for the prevention of disease and promotion of health. Today technical sophistication of modern medicine is not an answer to everyday common ailments of the vast poor in the country. Suitable technology and cheaper interventions such as Oral Rehydration Solution (ORS), immunization, etc are increasingly being applied as life saving measures and for disease prevention in society health care.

Doctors' role is no longer confined to diagnosing and treating those who come to the clinic. He is also responsible for those who need his service but cannot come to the clinic. Health of the people is not only the concern of healthcare providers. It is the duty of the society also to identify and solve their own health problems through their active participation.

All these changes in notion and concepts of health and healthcare system are embodied in society health care. The spate of new concepts and notions, for instance, increasing importance given to social justice and equity, recognition of vital role of society participation called for the new approaches to make medicine in the service of humanity more effective.

Alma-Ata declaration in 1978 specified that Primary Healthcare approach was the way of achieving the target of Health For All by 2000 AD. Primary Healthcare approach stressed that "essential healthcare ought to be made universally accessible to individuals and acceptable to them, through their full participation and at a cost the society and the country can afford".

## DEVELOPMENT OF PREVENTIVE AND SOCIAL MEDICINE

The Public Health administration in India actually commenced in 1869 with the appointment of a Sanitary Commission. The first Municipal Act was passed in 1884 in Bengal. However, in the Indian context J. P. Grant had visualised in 1939 that foreign models could not be suited for First Doctor Intervention or for Primary Health Care. His recommendations were also incorporated in Bhore Committee Report 1946, for building Community Doctors. The Bhore Committee's Report laid the foundation of modern public healthcare in India.

On the recommendations of Medical Education Conference in 1955, departments of Preventive and Social Medicine were established in Medical colleges all over the country. The experimental learning of our predecessors and Gurus provided the foundation and led to growth and expansion of the frontiers of the subject of Community Medicine. It has today evolved as a field of learning that contributes immensely to the progress and development of societies, more significantly in developing nations such as India. The professionals of Community Medicine have a main duty to shoulder i.e., to work for the health and well being of the people of India and contribute to education and production of basic physicians, well versed with handling community health problems. The target of medical education is to produce a basic physician who is competent to give complete healthcare to person, family and society. We need to bring about many changes, reforms in present medical education for achieving the desired target.

These departments have teaching/training, service and study constituents. But initially more emphasis was placed on teaching/training aspect. Beyond 1975, faculty members of Community Medicine were enriched with the field experiences in training, monitoring and assessment with active participation in several National Programmes such as ICDS (Integrated Child Development Scheme), EPI (Expanded Program on Immunization), UIP (Universal Immunization Program), CSSM (Child Survival and Safe Motherhood programme), NACP (National AIDS Control Program), RCH (Reproductive and Child Health programme) and have shared their experiences with the District/State/National Health Programme managers and also translated their experiences in Undergraduate and Postgraduate training and teaching.

There are variations in teaching/training in Preventive and Social Medicine in different states of India which reflects the cultural diversity and varying requirements of the local community. The study constituent has been a very poorly developed constituent of PSM so far mainly due to scarcity of funds.

Medical colleges have the primary function of imparting undergraduate medical education. These colleges form the majority of institutions in India, which render professional postgraduate qualification in Public Health. A school of public health such as All India Institute of Hygiene and Public Health, Calcutta, particularly established for the purpose without the duty of undergraduate medical education is an exception.

It is noted that many medical colleges are unable to have good community-oriented, field-based programmes for presentation and participatory education of the undergraduates. Medical colleges, by and large, remain isolated from healthcare system and play very limited role in public health services. However, desirable and positive changes through several approaches are taking place in the medical education system all over the world and in our country to enable it to stand upto the expectations of the country in the context of its overall social-economic-health development process e.g., by reorientation of curriculum, by community-based integrated teaching or by making medical colleges assume direct duty in rendering health care, etc.

The Government of India launched the Re-orientation of Medical Education scheme in the year 1977. The scheme aims at involving medical colleges directly in the healthcare delivery system by accepting total duty for promotive, preventive and curative healthcare of at least 3 Community Development Blocks in the first instance, ultimately extending to the whole district. The progress of the Scheme has been extremely slow in most colleges. There is hardly any impact on orienting medical students towards rural health care, which was its primary target. Medical graduates from most medical colleges still pass out with the same pattern of education, which was present earlier, with more focus on curative medicine and urban oriented approach. The healthcare system in India including medical education, healthcare services etc. as such, and not only Preventive and Social Medicine departments can be held responsible for this.

## CHALLENGES

In the field of Public Health & Preventive Medicine, tremendous changes have taken place, but greater changes can be anticipated in the coming decades. Concepts and policies cannot be static and planning must have sufficient flexibility to cope with the rapid-changing world of science and technology, of industrialization and urbanization.

It is obvious that new horizons and super-specialities are fast emerging in Preventive and Social Medicine, such as Epidemiology, MCH (Maternal and Child Health), IEC (Information Education Communication), Health Management, Health Economics, Nutrition, Demography, Health System Research, Environmental Health, etc. Present developments in Information Technology will certainly alter the face of Preventive and Social Medicine in the coming future.

Regular self-evaluation at a personal, institutional and at an association level is necessary. Newer roles and duties with ongoing 'strength, weakness, opportunities and threats' analysis can be identified. It will definitely help in further image building of the speciality in addition to improvement in health and overall development of the society.

There are many challenges in the field of Public Health. One of the challenges, which are successfully met, is "Eradication of Smallpox". This is a wonderful achievement which all of us are proud of. Other disease, which is successfully eliminated, is Guinea worm disease.

There were setbacks in some of the programmes such as Malaria, Tuberculosis that made us rethink and remodify the strategies and re-implement these national health programmes. As we are able to control some diseases, there will be new emerging as well re-emerging diseases. This faculty has to remain alert all the time and prepared for meeting the new challenges.

As per Charles Darwin, "It is not the strongest of the species that survive nor the most intelligent, but rather the one that is most responsive to change". Preventive and Social Medicine has demonstrated its survival instinct so far and will definitely acclimatise itself to changes in the society and emerge a winner.

## REFERENCES

Algranati PS. The pediatric patient: an approach to history and physical examination. Baltimore: Williams & Wilkins; 1992.

Coupey SM. Interviewing adolescents. Pediatr Clin North Am 1997; 44(6):1349-1364.

Ehram W, Matson S. Approach to assessing adolescents on serious or sensitive issues. Pediatr Clin North Am 1998; 45(1):189-204.

Elster A, Levenberg P. Integrating comprehensive adolescent preventive services into routine medical care. Pediatr Clin North Am 1997; 44(6):1365-1377.

Gill D, O'Brien N. Paediatric clinical examination, 3rd edn. London: Churchill Livingstone; 2000.

Ginsburg K. Guiding adolescents away from violence. Contemp Pediatr 1997; Goldenring JM, Cohen E. Getting into adolescent heads. Contemp Pediatr 1989; 5:75-90.

Hillard P. Preserving confidentiality in adolescent gynecology. Contemp Pediatr 1997; 14(6):71-92.

Knight J. Adolescent substance use: screening, assessment, and intervention. Contemp Pediatr 1997; 14(4):45-72.

Neinstein LS. Adolescent health care, 3rd edn. London: Williams & Wilkins; 1996.

Nicholson D, Ayers H. Adolescent problems: a practical guide for parents and teachers. London: David Fulton; 1997.

Orr D. Helping adolescents toward adulthood. Contemp Pediatr 1998; 15(5): 55-76.

Prazar G, Friedman S. An office-based approach to adolescent psychosocial issues. Contemp Pediatr 1997; 14(5):59-76.

Taylor J, Muller D. Nursing adolescents: research and psychological perspectives. Oxford: Blackwell Sciences; 1995.

Viner R. Youth matters. London: Action for Sick Children; 1999.

# 4

# Nursing Care of a Neonate

## ESSENTIAL NEWBORN CARE

Newborn nutrition is a vital part of the well-being of an infant. The stage of fast growth in infancy calls for careful nutritional support to continue the development and growth that started at conception. The first decision that parents need to make about feeding their infant is whether to breast-feed, bottle feed, or a combination of both. An early evaluation of feeding should have started during the first months of pregnancy. Nutritional information ought to be provided so that an informed decision can be made. It is significant that the parents know that there is a relationship between food and health. They ought to be given fundamental information about their infant's nutritional requirements and how they relate to breast milk, formula, or solid foods. After the baby is born, feeding practices ought to be examined, modified where essential, and reinforced. Proper nutrition is necessary for optimal development and growth of the newborn infant.

## NUTRITIONAL REQUIREMENTS OF THE NEWBORN

a. Fluid. Newborns require more fluid relative to their size than adults require. Extra fluids are needed with fever, diarrhoea, and vomiting.

   1. Dehydration. Till the ability to retain body water through kidney function improves in the early months of life, the infant is at risk for dehydration. Signs of dehydration are:

      a. Depressed fontanels.
      b. Fast, weak pulse.
      c. Elevated low-grade temperature.

d. Dark, concentrated urine.
e. Dry, hard stools.
f. Dry skin with little turgor.
g. Elevated specific gravity (1.020).

2. Water. Prepared infant formulas render enough water under usual environmental conditions. Water intoxication may result from excessive feeding of water to infants. It may occur when water is fed as a replacement for milk. Signs of water intoxication are:
   a. Hyponatremia.
   b. Weakness.
   c. Restlessness.
   d. Vomiting, diarrhoea.
   e. Polyuria or oliguria.
   f. Convulsions.
3. Nursing care.
   a. Preserve accurate input and output (I&O).
   b. Observe regularly for signs of dehydration or water intoxication.

b. Vitamin, Mineral, and Caloric Requirements.

- The newborn's fast growth makes him particularly vulnerable to dietary inadequacies and iron deficiency anaemia. Sufficient vitamin intake is particularly significant to support usual growth and metabolism. When the mother is well-nourished all through her pregnancy, the full-term neonate can be expected to have sufficient vitamin stores at birth. Calcium and iron are the two fundamental minerals that are of particular importance in maintaining sufficient nutrition.
- Calcium is necessary for the fast bone mineralization that takes place during the first year of life, muscle contraction, blood coagulation, nerve irritability, tooth development, and heart muscle action.
- Iron is a necessary element required for synthesis of haemoglobin and cell metabolism.
- Because of the limited nutritional stores, newborns require vitamin and mineral supplements. An infant may become hypoglycaemic and require feeding sooner than usual. His blood glucose is checked at one hour of age and if it is

decreased, the baby is first fed sips of water to ensure sucking swallowing coordination and is then fed formula to increase calories and decrease utilization of glucose.

## FIRST FEEDING FROM THE MOTHER

Signs of hunger are demonstrated by the infant searching for food, sucking motions, and crying. The mother may start to breast-feed at this time if she had planned to breast-feed, her condition is stable, and she desires to feed the infant.

## FORMULA FEEDINGS

a. Formula Requirements. A formula must fulfill the infant's requirements for water, calories, vitamins, and minerals. Commercially prepared formulas are made as per established standards.

b. Types of Formulas.

- Ready-to-feed. These are liquids packaged in cans and bottles. They are convenient and believed to be comparatively expensive.
- Concentrate. These are packaged in cans and are to be diluted 1:1 with water. This is less expensive.
- Powder. This must be mixed thoroughly with water and may have difficulty dissolving. This is believed to be the least expensive.

c. Formula Preparation in the Home.

- The choice of method is determined by the type of formula used, the safety of the home water supply, the availability of sufficient refrigeration, the ability to utilize the method, and the quantity of formula required each day.
- The aseptic method is used when preparing formula. Cleaning the equipment before preparing the formula is necessary. Formula is prepared as per directions and bottles assembled. As long as refrigeration is available, any number of bottles may be prepared.

d. Instructions for Feeding Formula.

- Formula at room temperature is usually well tolerated by the infant.
- Feeding should take place in a comfortable setting and in an unhurried manner.

- The newborn ought to be held in an elevated position. Bottles shouldn't be propped due to the danger of the choking and aspiration.
- An increased quantity of air may be sucked in if the infant is fed when lying flat.
- The bottle ought to be tilted to keep the nipple filled with milk/formula at all times.
- When the infant is held close during feedings, he gets more enjoyment from the security of being held by the parent or other person.
- Air bubbles can be seen going up into the bottle during feeding. This indicates that the baby is getting the formula.
- The infant must take at least one ounce every four hours.

e. Advantages of Formula Feeding.

- The mother can be sure the baby is getting sufficient milk for nutrition.
- There is an opportunity for other members of the family to get close to the baby. This allows the mother to give more of her time to her other children, to herself, or to her husband.

## BREAST-FEEDING

a. Preparation of the Nipples. Preparation of the nipples should start during pregnancy.

1. Roll nipples. The mother should roll her nipples with her thumb and forefinger two to three times each day.
2. Massage breast.
    - Place hand over the other above the breast.
    - Gently, but firmly, exert pressure evenly with the thumbs across the top and fingers underneath the breast.
    - Come together with the heel of the hand on each side and release at the areola, being careful not to touch the areola and nipple.
    - Gently lift the breast from beneath and drop lightly.

NOTE: The above procedure ought to be repeated 4 to 5 times with each breast.

3. Roughen nipples with a towel.

b. Initiation of Breast-feeding.

- Initial feeding is usually with one ounce of sterile water to determine if the newborn can swallow. The mother should start feeding with five minutes of actual sucking time on each breast and increase feeding time after the baby has fed three consecutive times without difficulty. Each feeding ought to be started by alternating the breasts. The baby may receive glucose water after feeding till the milk comes in the breast.
- The advantages of breast-feeding are as follows:
  - — Colostrum contains less fat and sugar and more protein and salts than breast milk. It also contains large quantities of antibodies and vitamins and acts as a laxative to help expel meconium.
  - — Protein is more digestible than cow's milk.
  - — The fat that is present is rich in essential fatty acids required for brain growth.
  - — Colostrum contains lactose, which favours the development of bacteria in the intestines that serves as a protective function during infancy.
  - — The calcium-to-phosphorous ratio is perfect for the absorption of calcium required for bone growth.
  - — It appears less likely to produce an obese child, promotes better tooth and jaw alignment, and protects against allergy development during infancy.
  - — Breast-feeding is convenient and eliminates formula preparation.
  - — Breast-feeding is economical.

c. Contraindications.

- Nipple or breast lesions may appear (depending upon the type).
- If the mother becomes pregnant, the milk will usually start to dry up.
- Maternal illness.
- Need of mother to return to work (though excellent battery operated breast pumps are now available and very inexpensive).
- Inability of the mother to psychologically adapt.
- A woman with cardiac or established renal disease may be discouraged from nursing.
- Infections.

d. Common Breast-Feeding Problems.

1. Delayed milk production. This is usually the earliest of breast-feeding problems. It occurs if the baby is not breast-fed within a short time after birth or not fed often enough.
2. Sore breasts.
   - The mother should let the baby breast-feed initially for ten to thirty minutes every two to three hours and bit by bit increase the quantity of time. If her breasts are not empty after feeding, have the mother to express the milk into a bottle and refrigerate for later feedings.
   - Improper position may cause soreness. Advise the mother that the infant should have a portion of the areola, in addition to the nipple in his mouth. Just chewing or sucking on the nipple may cause breast soreness.
3. Engorgement. This generally occurs on or about the third postpartum day. It results from an increase of milk into the milk ducts combined with increased blood and lymph supply to the breast. The breast becomes hard and painful. It is usually more common in the first-time breast-feeding mother. Engorgement can be prevented by:
   - Manual expression of milk if the breasts are full but the infant is not ready to nurse, or if the infant can not get hold of the nipple because the skin is too tight.
   - Wearing a supportive bra.
   - Frequent nursing, if not too painful.
   - Warm compresses applied to the sore breasts.

NOTE: The thumb and forefinger are placed on opposite sides of the breast just behind the areola. The lactiferous sinuses (ampulla A) are compressed, and milk is forced out.

4. Leaking breasts.
   - This is a common annoyance. A conditioned response will occur in the mother when she sees or hears a baby that causes the milk to let down.
   - The mother should fold her arms across her breasts and press them firmly against her chest wall. This will stop the leaking. Advise her to place absorbent pads in her bras.

5. Maternal anxiety. This will decrease milk production.
   a. An infant reacting to maternal anxiety will usually act in one of two ways.
   - He will suck, stop, cry, suck, stop, cry, and then may regurgitate.
   - He will suck, stop, cry, refuse to nurse, and continue to cry.

   b. Teach the mother relaxation techniques. Tell her to feed her baby in a quiet area.
6. Sore, cracked, or fissured nipples.
   a. Causes.
   1. Infant not having the nipple and areola properly in the mouth.
   2. "Friction" of the baby's gums on the nipple.
   3. Infant being allowed to suck on an empty breast.
   4. Washing the nipples with soap, which is drying.
   5. Failure to break suction before removing the infant from the breast.

   b. Nursing interventions. Teach the mother proper nursing techniques and proper breast care.
7. Breast infection.
   - Most frequently caused by the causative organism, Staphylococcus areus.
   - Entry is gained through a cracked or fissured nipple.
   - The infection is usually interstitial and not intraductal, so the infections will not harm the baby.
   - Nursing interventions. Instruct the mother on proper breast care. If breast soreness is present, have the mother to express milk into a bottle to feed to her baby.

## BUBBLING THE NEWBORN

- Methods used to bubble the baby are baby placed on shoulders, baby held upright leaning slightly forward, and baby held across the lap. Rub or gently pat his back till air is expelled.
- When no belch follows feeding, position the baby on his right side or abdomen.

c. The baby ought to be bubbled regularly.
   - Bottle-feeding-every 1/2 ounce initially.
   - Breast-feeding-between each breast.

d. Always be sure to support the head.

## ASSESSING NUTRITIONAL STATUS

a. Observe.

- Behaviour (crying, content, short sleeper).
- Measure either fluid intake from bottle fed newborn or number of minutes at each breast.
- Watch for signs of dehydration.
- Daily weights (assess increases and decreases).
- Elimination pattern.
  - — Dark, concentrated urine means too little fluid intake.
  - — Hard stools mean too little fluid intake.
  - — Frequency of stools or urine.
- Low-grade temperatures and/or increasing, weak pulses.

b. Determine impact of the observations over a 24-hour period rather than at each feeding.

## WEIGHT CHANGES

- All babies lose weight directly after birth, which should cause no concern unless the weight loss approaches 10 percent of the birth weight.
- Within a week a newborn should regain his birth weight.
- A gain of about an ounce a day is average.
- At the end of 5 months, most babies have doubled their birth weight.

## FIRST ORAL FEEDING AND RECORDING PROCEDURES BY THE NURSE

- Review the mother's health record to verify the order.
- Wash the hands.
- Assemble the essential equipment (sterile water in bottle, nipple and cap combination, tissue or cloth, and gown if essential).
- Wash the hands.
- Put on clean gown (if not already in scrubs).
- Approach and identify the newborn.
- Invert the bottle and shake some water on the wrist.
  - — Test the potency of the nipple hole.
  - — Ensure that the water drips freely, but not in a stream. If the hole is too large, the newborn may aspirate water.

If the hole is too small, the newborn may tire before the end of feeding.

- Sit comfortable and cradle the newborn in a semi-reclining position in one arm. The infant's head and back are easily supported. Air is allowed to rise to the top of the infant's stomach where it is more easily expelled.
- Place the nipple in the newborn's mouth. Don't insert if far enough to stimulate a gag reflex. The newborn should start to suck. If he does not, stroke him under the chin or on the side of his cheek, or touch his lips with the nipple to stimulate a sucking reflex.
- Tilt the bottle upward as the newborn feeds. Keep the nipple filled with water. This prevents him from swallowing air. Watch for a steady stream of bubbles in the bottle. This indicates proper venting and flow of water.
- Reinsert the nipple if the newborn pushes the nipple out with his tongue. This is a usual reflex. It doesn't necessarily mean that he is finished eating.
- Burp (bubble) the newborn after each 1/2 ounces of water. Some air will be swallowed by the newborn even when fed properly. Positions to bubble the newborn are:
  - Hold the newborn upright in a slightly forward position. Use one hand to support his head and cheek. Rub or gently pat his back till air is expelled.
  - Hold the newborn upright over the shoulder or place him face down across the lap. A change in position helps bring up the bubble. Rub or gently pat his back till air is expelled.
- Place the newborn on his stomach or right side. This prevents aspiration if he regurgitates.
- Discard any remaining formula and correctly dispose of all equipment.
- Record the procedures and important nursing observations in the patient's health record. Give the same report to the Charge Nurse. This will include:
  - Time of feeding.
  - Quantity taken.
  - How well the newborn fed.

— Did neonate appear satisfied.

— Occurrence of any regurgitation or vomiting.

## FORMULA PREPARATION INSTRUCTIONS TO THE MOTHER

Reinforce instruction to the mother about formula preparation.

- Identify the mother requiring reinforcement of teaching.
- Review the mother's records to identify information previously given.
  — Facts about formula preparation and storage.
  — Facts about feeding equipment.
- Formula preparation and storage.

1. Commercially prepared formulas ought to be stored in cool places till opened. Once opened, the formula ought to be refrigerated at temperature and times suggested by the manufacturer.
   — Once formula (or powder) has been constituted with water, follow the manufacturer's suggestions for length of time constituted formula is good.
   — Once the newborn starts to feed, constituted formula ought to be used within 30 minutes. If not discarded, formula serves as an excellent medium for bacterial growth.
2. Formulas prepared in the home ought to be stored in the refrigerator after the initial cool-down period following sterilization.
   — Bottles of formula that have been sterilized are believed to be "good" till opened.
   — Once opened, these bottles ought to be used within 30 minutes time frame. The unused portion ought to be discarded and not saved for the next feeding.
3. Ready-to-feed formulas ought to be stored in a cool place. Once opened, these feedings ought to be used within 30 minutes and not saved for subsequent feedings.
4. Dilution of formulas is of extreme importance. Improper dilution may cause problems like diarrhoea (if too concentrated) and weight loss (if too dilute).

## FEEDING EQUIPMENT

1. Bottles.
   — May be sterilized at home.
   — May be cleansed by meticulous washing with warm, sudsy water and rinsing in hot water, and then air-dried.
   — Plastic bottle inserts may be used but ought to be discarded after each use. The folds of plastic around the junction of the bottle's neck and the nipple render a good source of growth medium.
   — Ready-to-feed bottles pre-filled with formula may be purchased but are quite expensive.

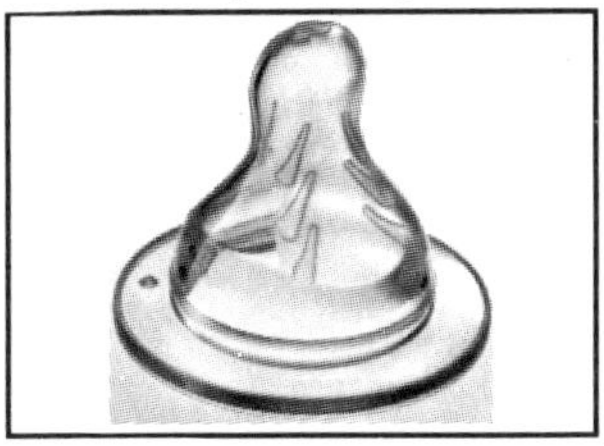

*Fig. Feeding Equipment*

2. Nipples may be meticulously cleansed at home or may be purchased as a nipple-cap combination.
   - Clarify the mother's understanding of initial instructions.
     — Render information to correct any misunderstanding.
     — Refer any questions the parents can't answer to the Charge Nurse.
   - Render extra instruction, as essential, to the mother.
   - Determine the mother's understanding by questioning key points.
   - Report and record the mother's instruction suitably.

## NEONATAL RESUSCITATION

Neonatology, perinatology and neonatal resuscitation developed to a great extent during the 1970's in response to an epidemic of litigation involving birth brain injury; foetal monitoring was detecting foetal distress in utero, and specialized perinatal intensive care promised great improvement in neonatal morbidity and mortality. Today, in hospitals, if a child is born alive, the chances of it dying within a few days are virtually zero; even some babies without a heartbeat are resuscitated. Perhaps one third of all neonates receive some form of resuscitation treatment, and the success in terms of mortality is excellent. About 6% to 10% of all neonates are "morbid" and need NICU care - many of these are preemies; again, NICU mortality is extremely rare; however, in terms of neurological and mental disability, particularly in NICU babies, long-term morbidity is anything but rare. The life-saving procedures of neonatal resuscitation and NICU care are much less successful in preserving brains. If resuscitation doesn't result in a five minute Apgar of 7 or more, neurological impairment is likely.

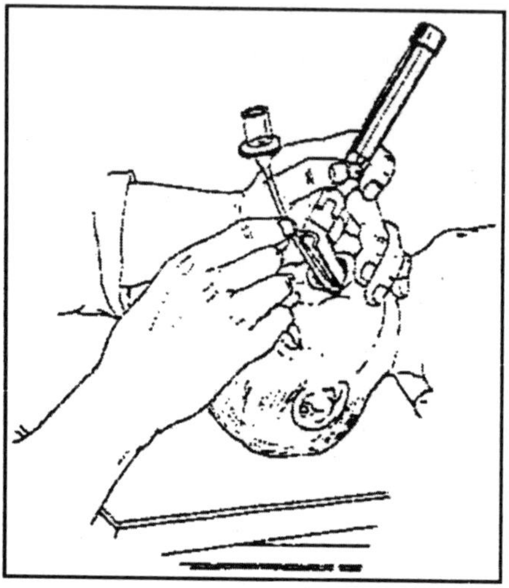

*Fig. Neonatal Resuscitation*

The term "resuscitation" implies restoration of deficient life support systems, particularly respiration; in the depressed newborn, that inadequacy is in the placenta and cord, as the lungs have not yet begun to function. The rationale on which current resuscitation is based is that early detection of foetal asphyxia combined with fast delivery and fast establishment of pulmonary respiration (reversal of asphyxia) will prevent brain injury.

If brain damage (neuron necrosis) has occurred in utero, resuscitation will not heal it; however, overt brain damage seldom is apparent at birth, and it frequently appears after resuscitation. Hypoxic ischemic encephalopathy usually is diagnosed hours after birth when the child convulses; germinal matrix haemorrhage in preemies may develop a day or two after birth; mental and behavioural problems may not surface for years.

The normal consensus is that birth "asphyxia" is the cause of the brain damage; hypoxia is a more precise term, though asphyxia implies inhibition of respiration - respiration includes oxygen supply and removal of carbon dioxide. Iatrogenic resuscitation usually corrects this asphyxia promptly by initiating pulmonary ventilation; most organs survive superbly, all except the brain. This strongly implies that there are other factors active in neonatal "depression" besides hypoxia and acidosis that must be corrected during "resuscitation". The placenta is much more than a respiratory organ. Correction of the placental/cord inadequacy that caused the depression, and support of placental function are thus rational priorities in revival of a depressed neonate, just as they are in the "resuscitation" of the "distressed" foetus in utero.

In utero, the general blood supply of the foetal brain is comparatively hypoxic. Umbilical vein blood is fairly well oxygenated, but it is mixed in the inferior vena cava and in the heart with de-oxygenated blood from the venae cavae; this is then circulated systemically. The colour of a normal newborn is purple - it has been purple for nine months - circulating a mixture of haemoglobin (blue) and oxyhaemoglobin (red). It turns pink only after the foetal circulation is changed to the adult circulation, and is combined with aeration of the lungs.

The foetal brain thus grows and develops with a copious blood supply that is only partially oxygenated, but which readily removes products of aerobic and anaerobic respiration and excretes them through the placenta. The foetal kidneys and gut thrive on blood with the same oxygen partial pressure as the blood flowing to the placenta to be oxygenated. The newborn brain and other organs are consequently comparatively immune to pure hypoxic injury as long as organ and placental perfusion are copious.

The same fundamental principles apply to the adult brain; five minutes or more of cardiac arrest will produce some brain damage or brain death; occlusion of a cerebral artery rapidly results in infarction (death) of the supplied tissue. On the other hand, five minutes or more of pure anoxia (e.g. breathing pure nitrogen) will produce unconsciousness that is fully reversible without brain damage provided that brain perfusion is not impaired. The integrity of the newborn brain is maintained (by perfusion and oxygenation) at usual (physiological) birth; consequently the physiological mechanisms that ensure these functions (perfusion and oxygenation) ought to be supported and/or duplicated during iatrogenic resuscitation if brain damage is to be avoided.

The critically depressed/asphyxiated newborn typically shows not only no sign of breathing, but also lack of muscle tone and reflexes required to start breathing, in addition to signs of hypoxia like cyanosis;

in the most severe cases, pallor indicates vasomotor collapse. Such a child has obviously suffered a main respiratory insult prior to or during birth; the cause of that insult and its particular effects are factors that must be corrected, if possible, in the resuscitation process.

In any and every case of newborn depression, if a child is born alive - with a heart beat and a pulsating cord - the placental life support system has not failed completely; utilization of this system in resuscitation and transition to "adult" life support systems in the depressed newborn is necessary in restoring the physiological state - health - without the incursion of organ damage, primary or secondary, from "birth asphyxia." With early detection of foetal distress and with fast delivery, the neonate's central nervous system ought to be undamaged at birth; the target of therapy ought to be that it remains so.

## NORMAL (PHYSIOLOGICAL) RESUSCITATION AT BIRTH - TRANSITION

At normal (physiological) birth, the child "resuscitates" itself:

- Its wet, cooling skin triggers the "cold crying reflex" and "cold pressor reflex."
- The foetal circulation is switched to the adult circulation.
- The lungs are aerated, and the umbilical vessels then close reflexively.

There is no period of asphyxia or hypo-perfusion. However, this description is very simplistic and incomplete.

The switch from placental to lung "breathing" is only a portion of the whole; the switch from placental alimentation and placental excretion to the newborn's alimentary and excretory organs is also part of "natural" resuscitation. To start and establish the newborn functions of the lungs, gut, kidneys, and other systems, including the brain, continuous copious perfusion of these organs is needed; a large transfusion of placental blood during natural childbirth "resuscitates," or more properly "activates" all these organ systems as the massive flow of blood through the placenta (40% of the foetal cardiac output) is diverted to these organs during physiological closure of the cord vessels.

Cord closure abruptly halts the placental supply of glucose to the brain (used in aerobic and anaerobic respiration); the neonatal liver (glycogen stores) must start to maintain blood glucose levels. A major portion of the liver's blood supply is from the hepatic portal vein that derives its blood from the mesenteric arteries. If the gut (and hence the liver) is not "copiously perfused," hypoglycemia may result in a neonatal convulsion. Deficient perfusion of the liver may also be a factor in bilirubin excretion and "physiological" jaundice.

Copious perfusion of the neonatal kidneys with sufficient blood pressure is needed for solute excretion, fluid, electrolyte and acid-base regulation after the placenta ceases to function.

During the third stage of labour while the cord is pulsating, warm blood from the placenta courses through the newborn. After cord closure, temperature regulation is abruptly needed of the neonate; switch of blood flow to and from the epidermis calls for a copious quantity of blood to influence heat loss and heat retention.

In the faetus, pulmonary circulation is minimal; after the adult circulation is established, the total cardiac output flows through the lungs. A major portion of the placental transfusion is utilized in establishing pulmonary blood flow after birth. Jaykka demonstrated that perfusion of the foetal lung "erected" the alveoli and actually started aeration; the high colloid osmotic pressure of the circulating blood rapidly absorbs amniotic fluid from the erected alveoli. Thus sufficient "copious perfusion" of the lungs may result in pulmonary oxygenation before any muscular respiratory effort occurs.

Respiratory effort is reflexively controlled through the central nervous system; hypoxia and increased concentration of carbon dioxide are strong stimulants for receptors. For the reflex to function, copious perfusion of the reflex circuit is needed, as is copious perfusion of the respiratory muscles.

An extra factor in "normal" resuscitation/transition is increased systemic blood pressure caused by placental transfusion, the cold pressor reflex and closure of the umbilical arteries; this may reverse blood flow in the ductus arteriosus and increase "erection" of lung tissue. Increased blood pressure also increases glomerular filtration in the kidneys and causes increased fluid loss into the extra-cellular space ensuing in haemo-concentration. The consequent increase in plasma colloid osmotic pressure prevents pulmonary oedema and dries up the lungs. Thus natural "resuscitation" is the physiological switch from the placental life support system to all the independent corresponding organ systems of the newborn; it involves much more than ventilation of the lungs. The most significant factor is the placental transfusion that increases the newborn's blood volume by 30% to 50%, the extra blood being utilized to activate and establish the functioning of these organ systems. Comprehension of this physiology is necessary for elucidating the factors in neonatal depression and in iatrogenic resuscitation that produce the variety of pathology seen in the NICU following incomplete recuperation of the depressed newborn.

## IATROGENIC RESUSCITATION

The routine procedure for resuscitating an "at risk" or depressed newborn is prompt clamping of the umbilical cord followed by transfer to a warmer where the child's airway is cleared (by visualization of the vocal cords and tracheal suction in cases of meconium staining) and the baby is stimulated by rubbing the skin. If respiration doesn't occur within 30 seconds or so, bag-mask ventilation is commenced; if this fails to produce spontaneous respiration, endo-tracheal intubation is performed with positive pressure ventilation.

Prompt cord clamping produces the major deviations from "natural resuscitation"; placental oxygenation, placental acidosis regulation, placental glucose supply and placental transfusion are all abruptly aborted and the child is subjected to a stage of complete asphyxiation till the lungs function. The warmer deprives the child of the cold crying and cold pressor reflexes. Bag-masking or intubation ventilation readily aerates the alveoli; this reflexively dilates pulmonary arterioles and promotes pulmonary perfusion and the switch from foetal to adult circulation; however, without additional blood volume that is generally supplied by placental transfusion, less than optimal pulmonary perfusion may occur ensuing in less than optimal gas exchange and incomplete closure of the foramen ovale and the ductus arteriosus.

The promptly clamped newborn has, in effect, been subjected to a massive haemorrhage, losing up to 50% of its blood volume; however, the actual quantity of blood loss varies greatly with the circumstances of the particular birth and with the speed with which the cord is clamped. At normal, spontaneous delivery, the contracting uterus may squeeze blood into the child during the second stage of labour; if the child cries before the trunk is delivered, the contraction that delivers the child may also deliver a "full" placental transfusion before the clamp can be applied. Likewise, a mother who delivers in the squatting position will usually transfuse the child fairly sufficiently by gravity before the clamp can be applied. A usual, spontaneous delivery (with the mother supine) followed by prompt placement of the child on the mother's abdomen may result in considerable gravitational blood loss into the placenta if the clamp is placed during uterine diastole. Rarely, when a clamp happens to be placed during a strong uterine contraction, the child may be over-transfused with blood that would have drained back into the placenta had the clamp not been placed. Generally, most newborns that breathe promptly after a usual vaginal delivery will not lose a critical quantity of blood volume from early cord clamping.

This, no doubt, has led to complacency about prompt cord clamping; however, many promptly clamped newborns, particularly those that are apneic, have much less than an optimal blood volume, and some are very blood volume deficient. After a "normal" birth and prompt cord clamping, they may develop infant anaemia months later, and years later, in grade school, they may be found to be mentally deficient.

The apneic child that is delivered above the level of the placenta that is in a relaxed uterus will suffer gravitational blood loss into the placenta. This fact is used as rationale for prompt clamping at cesarean section. The procedure certainly prevents prompt newborn blood loss, but the sectioned child thus delivered is routinely hypovolemic from loss of placental transfusion. Sectioned newborns have a higher incidence of RDS and persistent foetal circulation (PFC) than do vaginal deliveries; Landau completely prevented RDS in sectioned babies by leaving the placenta attached and suspending it above the child such as an I.V. An important number of perfectly normal, term babies die from PFC following elective c-section.

Premature babies are routinely promptly clamped for transfer to resuscitation. The premature placenta is comparatively large in relation to the faetus and contains a correspondingly larger portion of the feto-placental blood volume. The blood loss from immediate clamping is, consequently, correspondingly greater. All such preemies develop anaemia. Shock lung (RDS/hyaline membrane disease [HMD]) is a common complication. Kinmond prevented RDS in preemies by gravitational placental transfusion and also eliminated the need for red cell transfusion. The routine use of physiological cord closure has NEVER been reported; there are many indications that such preemies would be healthier than those of Kinmond. In the extremely immature infant, preservation of the placental circulation with immersion of the placenta in a suitable nutrient medium would appear to be rational therapy to support the immature life support systems. RDS and HMD are readily produced in newborn foals by immediate cord clamping and in newborn rabbits and puppies by removal of blood volume. It would appear that sufficient blood volume at birth is necessary for usual lung function. RDS/HMD from hypovolemia may occur at any age regardless of the presence or absence of surfactant in the lungs.

The most common cause of foetal distress in labour is cord compression (cord around the neck, cord prolapse, knot in the cord, oligohydramnios), and measures to relieve cord compression (re-positioning the patient, amnio-infusion, elevation of the presenting part, stopping labour with uterine relaxants) may succeed in returning the foetal heart tracing to normal - may resuscitate the faetus. If these measures don't succeed, the child is born "depressed," its cord is clamped immediately, and it is transferred to the resuscitation table. Intra-partum cord compression impedes cord venous blood flow (oxygenated, non-acidotic) to the child while allowing cord arterial flow (high pressure) to engorge the placenta. Thus the very "depressed" child (following cord compression) is born in hypovolemic shock, complicated by hypoxia and acidosis - limp and pallid. Immediate cord clamping seals its fate.

If the cord is not clamped and the compression is relieved, (knot loosened, cord unwound from the neck) and the child is lowered, blood drains from the engorged placenta into the child and the hypovolemic, hypoxic shock is reversed within 30 seconds with transfusion of oxygenated, non-acidotic blood; placental respiration reverses the "depression." This third stage therapy mimics successful intra-uterine resuscitation.

If the cord compression has been of some duration ("intra-uterine asphyxia," Linderkamp), e.g. oligohydramnios, the high hydrostatic pressure in the placental capillaries may have dehydrated the faetus, causing marked haemoconcentration. This situation is frequently reversed in utero by amnioinfusion; if it is not corrected, the immediately clamped neonate is prone to develop the "hyper-viscosity syndrome," a combination of dehydration, hypovolemia and haemoconcentration. While placental circulation and placental transfusion (delayed clamping) may assist in this situation, in the more severe cases, the cord vessels are constricted and little placental blood is available; intravenous hydration may also be required to restore physiology.

In asphyxia caused by placental abruption, increase in carbon dioxide may dilate placental and cord vessels, causing a shift in blood volume from the faetus; in the pre-term faetus, the more premature the child, the higher is the placental portion of the feto-placental blood volume. In nearly all "risk" deliveries subjected to immediate cord clamping, there is strong potential for severe hypovolemia at birth.

The neonate reacts to hypovolemia with massive generalized vaso-constriction that shifts volume circulation from less vital organs to the heart and brain. Depending upon the degree of hypovolemia, the clinical signs vary from weakness to those of hypovolemic shock: pallor, hypotension, hypothermia, oliguria/anuria, metabolic acidosis, anaemia and respiratory distress syndrome (RDS) otherwise known as "shock lung." Hypoglycemia caused by deficient liver perfusion has already been mentioned. They are seldom recognized for what they are, because neonatologists are indoctrinated with the notion that placental transfusion is a pathological event and that an immediately clamped newborn has a normal blood volume. Many neonatologists have never seen a newborn that has closed its cord physiologically.

There are many consequences of this conceptual error - the inadequate and tardy use of blood volume expanders and blood transfusion in ischemic encephalopathy; the use of medication (vasoconstrictors) to maintain blood pressure in hypovolemic shock while vasoconstriction is causing oliguria and ischemic necrosis of the bowel - necrotizing entero-colitis; the use of surfactant to treat RDS (shock lung) while the hypovolemic shock remains untreated and lungs are under-perfused. All of these and other consequences, and particularly those consequences relating to brain damage, become irrelevant when the conceptual error is corrected and rational management of neonatal depression is employed.

## NURSING MANAGEMENT OF A LOW BIRTH WEIGHT BABY

Nurses have a vital role in the successful operation and ultimate outcome of low birth weight babies' care and therapy. Neonatal intensive care nursing is the highly specialised area of knowledge and practice that calls for lengthy supervised experience to reach a level of competence that permits independent nursing care. It involves an understanding of neonatal physiology and characteristic knowledge of the function and management of a number of mechanical devices and apparatus, the ability to recognise very subtle deviation from the expected and the ability in implementing a judicious course of action.

Birth weight is regarded as a major determinant of neonatal death in the developing world. As per W.H.O., new borns with birth weight of 2500 gms or less ought to be designated as low birth weight babies. It was assessed by Indian scientists that 2000 gms or less ought to be taken as the criteria for low birth weight of Indian infants. It was found to be 5.5 % as against 20-30% when the criteria was less than 2500 gms. The term very low birth weight refers to weight between 1000 gms to 1500 gms regardless of gestational age. Out of 22 million low birth infants in the world, 21 million belongs to developing countries. India shows quite substantial 7-10 million low birth weights constituting 30% of all the birth in India. The reason for having such a high prevalence may be because of illiteracy, poverty, insufficient antenatal care, maternal nutritional deficits and high parity.

The main findings are as follows:

- Incidence of low birth weight is higher amongst mothers not receiving regular antenatal care.
- Systemic Diseases like anaemia, pre-echmpsia [PET], Hepatitis during pregnancy is direct contributory factors to increased incidence of low birth weight babies.
- Primigravida and grand multi-para were more prone to deliver low birth weight babies.
- Incidence of low birth weight babies is higher in the mothers from poor socio-economic status.
- Major neonatal complication in low birth weight babies are respiratory distress, Jaundice, Birth asphyxia, Pneumonia and septicaemia.
- Low birth babies require unique care like ventilation, U.V. phototherapy, Nebulization and oxygen administration in accordance with complication.
- All low birth babies require suctioning and oxygen therapy by nasal catheter placed in front of nostrils (Free flow oxygen).
- Body temperature of all babies ought to be maintained by over head warmer in the labour room.

## RECOMMENDATIONS

- All antenatal women should receive regular antenatal care.
- High-risk antenatal mothers like cases of PET, malnutrition, anaemia etc. ought to be screened early and directed towards hospital for safe delivery.
- Health education programme ought to be conducted for antenatal mothers regarding factors contributing to low birth weight.
- Nurses ought to be well oriented and trained to handle the equipments.

- Each P.H.C. ought to be provided with life saving equipments like oxygen, suction apparatus, heaters, ambu bags etc.
- In-service education ought to be conducted for staff nurses regarding care of LBW babies and use of mechanical devices.

## KANGAROO MOTHER CARE

Kangaroo mother care is a method of care of preterm infants which involves infants being carried, usually by the mother, with skin-to-skin contact. This guide is intended for health professional responsible for the care of low-birth-weight and preterm infants. Designed to be adapted to local conditions, it provides guidance on how to organize services at the referral level and on what is required to render effective kangaroo mother care.

The guide provides practical advice on when and how the Kangaroo Mother Care (KMC) method can best be applied. It is intended for health professionals caring for low-birth-weight and pre-term newborn babies in first referral hospitals with scarce resources. It also provides decision-makers and planners at the national and local levels with necessary information for deciding on the appropriateness of KMC for their health system and identifying what is needed to implement it successfully.

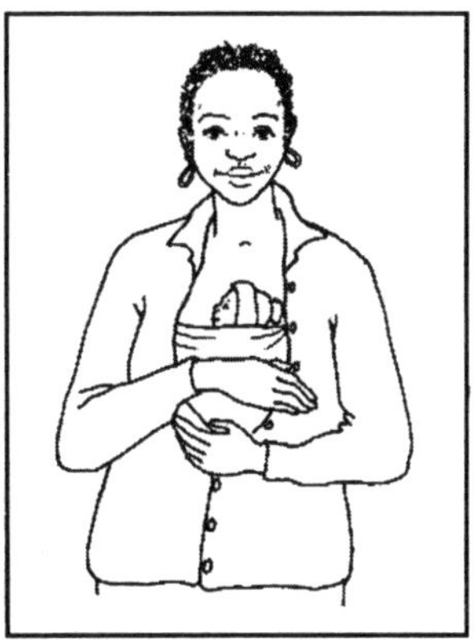

*Fig. Kangaroo Mother Care*

Some 20 million low-birth-weight (LBW) babies are born each year, due to either preterm birth or impaired prenatal growth, mostly in less developed countries. They contribute substantially to a high rate of neonatal mortality whose frequency and distribution correspond to those of poverty.1, 2 LBW and preterm birth are thus linked with high neonatal and infant mortality and morbidity.3, 4 Of the estimated 4 million neonatal deaths, preterm and LBW babies represent more than a fifth.5 Consequently, the care of such infants becomes a burden for health and social systems everywhere.

In affluent societies the major contributor to LBW is preterm birth. The rate has been decreasing thanks to improved socioeconomic conditions, lifestyles and nutrition, ensuing in healthier pregnancies, and to modern neonatal care technology and highly specialised and skilled health workers.

In less developed countries high rates of LBW are because of preterm birth and impaired intrauterine growth, and their prevalence is decreasing slowly. Because reasons and determinants remain largely unknown, effective interventions are limited. Moreover, modern technology is either not available or can't be used correctly, frequently because of the shortage of skilled staff. Incubators, for example, where available, are frequently inadequate to meet local requirements or are not sufficiently cleaned. Purchase of the equipment and spare parts, maintenance and repairs are difficult and costly; the power supply is intermittent, so the equipment doesn't work correctly. Under such circumstances good care of preterm and LBW babies is difficult: hypothermia and nosocomial infections are frequent, aggravating the poor outcomes because of prematurity. Often and frequently unnecessarily, incubators separate babies from their mothers, depriving them of the essential contact.

Unfortunately, there is no simple solution to this problem because the health of an infant is closely associated to the mother's health and the care she receives in pregnancy and childbirth. For many small preterm infants, receiving prolonged medical care is significant. However, kangaroo mother care (KMC) is an effective way to meet baby's requirements for warmth, breastfeeding, protection from infections, stimulation, safety and well being.

Kangaroo Mother Care (KMC) is a unique way of caring of low birth weight babies. It fosters their health and well being by promoting effective thermal control, breastfeeding, infection prevention and bonding. In KMC, the baby is continuously kept in skin-to-skin contact by the mother and breastfed exclusively to the extreme extent, KMC is started in the hospital and continued at home.

## COMPONENTS OF KANGAROO MOTHER CARE

The two components of KMC are:

- Skin-to-skin contact: Early, continuous and prolonged skin-to-skin contact between the mother and her baby is the fundamental component of KMC. The infant is placed on her mother's chest between the breasts.

- Exclusive breastfeeding: The baby on KMC is breastfed exclusively. Skin-to-skin contact promotes lactation and facilitates the feeding interaction.

## PRE-REQUISITES OF KMC

The two pre-requisites of KMC are:

- Support to the mother in hospital and at home A mother can't successfully render KMC all alone. She would require counselling along with supervision from care-providers, and assistance and cooperation from her family members. Skin to skin contact of the infant on the mother's chest
- Post-discharge follow up KMC is continued at home after early discharge from the hospital. A regular follow up and access to health providers for solving problem are vital to ensure safe and successful KMC at home.

## BENEFITS OF KMC

- Breastfeeding: Researches have revealed that KMC results in increased breastfeeding rates in addition to increased duration of breastfeeding. Even when started late and for a limited time during day and night, KMC has been shown to exert a useful effect on breastfeeding.
- Thermal control: Prolonged skin-to-skin contact between the mother and her preterm/LBW infant provides effective thermal control with a reduced risk of hypothermia. For stable babies, KMC is at least equivalent to conventional care with incubators in terms of safety and thermal protection.
- Early discharge: Researches have shown that KMC cared LBW infants could be discharged from the hospital earlier than the conventionally managed babies. The babies gained more weight on KMC than on conventional care.
- Less morbidity: Babies receiving KMC have more regular breathing and less predisposition to apnea. KMC protects against nosocomial infections. Even after discharge from the hospital, the morbidity amongst babies managed by KMC is less. KMC is linked with reduced incidence of severe illness including pneumonia during infancy.

- Other effects: KMC helps both infants and parents. Mothers are less stressed during kangaroo care as compared with a baby kept in incubator. Mothers prefer skin-to-skin contact to conventional care. They report a stronger bonding with the baby, increased confidence, and a deep satisfaction that they were able to do something unique for their babies. Fathers felt more relaxed, comfortable and better bonded while rendering kangaroo care.

## REQUIREMENTS FOR KMC IMPLEMENTATION

- Training of nurses, doctors and other staff involved in the care of the mother and the baby.
- Educational material like information sheets, posters, video films on KMC in local language ought to be available to the mothers, families and society.
- If possible, reclining chairs in the nursery and postnatal wards, and beds with adjustable back rest ought to be arranged. Mother can render KMC sitting on an ordinary chair or in a semi-reclining posture on a bed with the assistance of pillows.

## ELIGIBILITY CRITERIA

### Baby

All stable LBW babies are eligible for KMC. However, very sick babies needing unique care ought to be cared under radiant warmer initially. KMC ought to be commenced after the baby is haemo-dynamically stable. Guidelines for practicing KMC include:

- Birth weight >1800 g: These babies are in general stable at birth. Consequently, in most of them KMC can be started soon after birth.
- Birth weight 1200-1799 g: Many babies of this group have important problems in neonatal stage. It might take a few days before KMC can be started. If such a baby is born in a place where neonatal care services are insufficient, he ought to be transferred to a proper facility promptly after birth, along with the mother/family member. He ought to be transferred to a referral hospital after initial stabilization and suitable management; one of the best ways of transporting small babies is by keeping them in continuous skin-to-skin contact with the mother/family member during transport.

- Birth weight <1200 g: Often, these babies develop serious prematurity-related morbidity frequently starting soon after birth. They benefit the most from in-utero transfer to the institutions with neonatal intensive care facilities. It may take days to weeks before baby's condition allows initiation of KMC.

## Mother

All mothers can render KMC, irrespective of age, parity, education, culture and religion. The following points must be taken into consideration when counselling on KMC:

- Willingness: The mother must be willing to render KMC. Healthcare providers should counsel and motivate her. Once the mother realises the benefits of KMC for her baby, she will learn and undertake KMC.
- General health and nutrition: The mother ought to be free from serious illness to be able to render KMC. She should receive sufficient diet and supplements suggested by her doctor.
- Hygiene: The mother should maintain good hygiene: daily bath/ sponge, change of clothes, hand washing, short and clean finger nails.
- Supportive family: Apart from supporting the mother, family members should also be encouraged to render KMC when mother wishes to take rest. Mother would need family's cooperation to deal with her conventional duties of household chores until the baby requires KMC.
- Supportive community: Community awareness about the benefits ought to be produced. This is especially significant when there are social, economic or family constraints.

## PREPARING FOR KMC

When baby is ready for KMC, arrange a time that is convenient to the mother and her baby. The first few sessions are significant and require extended interaction. Demonstrate to her the KMC procedure in a caring, gentle manner and with patience. Answer her queries and allay her anxieties. Encourage her to bring her mother/mother in law, husband or any other member of the family. It assists in building positive attitude of the family and ensuring family support to the mother which is especially vital for post-discharge home-based KMC. It is useful that the mother starting KMC, interacts with someone already practicing KMC for her baby.

## MOTHER'S CLOTHING

KMC can be provided using any front-open, light dress according to the local culture. KMC works well with blouse and sari, gown or shawl. An appropriate apparel that can retain the baby for extended stage of time can be adapted locally.

### Baby's Clothing

Baby is dressed with cap, socks, nappy, and front-open sleeveless shirt or 'jhabala'.

## THE KMC PROCEDURE

### Kangaroo Positioning

- The baby ought to be placed between the mother's breasts in an upright position.
- The head ought to be turned to one side and in a slightly extended position. This slightly extended head position keeps the airway open and allows eye to eye contact between the mother and her baby.
- The hips ought to be flexed and abducted in a "frog" position; the arms should also be flexed.
- Baby's abdomen ought to be at the level of the mother's epigastrium. Mother's breathing stimulates the baby, thus reducing the occurrence of apnea.
- Support the baby's bottom with a sling/binder.

### Monitoring

Babies receiving KMC ought to be monitored carefully particularly during the initial stages. Nursing staff should make sure that baby's neck position is neither too flexed nor too extended, airway is clear, breathing is regular, colour is pink and baby is maintaining temperature. Mother ought to be involved in observing the baby during KMC so that she herself can continue monitoring at home.

### Feeding

The mother ought to be explained how to breastfeed while the baby is in KMC position. Holding the baby near the breast stimulates milk production. She may express milk while the baby is still in KMC position. The baby could be fed with paladai, spoon or tube, depending upon the condition of the baby.

## Privacy

KMC unavoidably calls for some exposure on the part of the mother. This can make her nervous and could be de-motivating. The staff must respect mother's sensitivities in this regard and ensure culturally-acceptable privacy standards in the nursery and the wards where KMC is practiced.

## Time of Initiation

KMC can be commenced as soon as the baby is stable. Babies with severe illnesses or requiring unique treatment ought to be managed as per the unit protocol. Short KMC sessions can be started during recuperation with ongoing medical treatment (IV fluids, oxygen therapy). KMC can be provided while the baby is being fed via orogastric tube or on oxygen therapy.

## Duration of KMC

- Skin-to-skin contact should begun gradually in the nursery, with a smooth transition from conventional care to continuous KMC.
- Sessions that last less than one hour ought to be avoided because frequent handling may be stressful for the baby.
- The length of skin-to-skin contacts ought to be gradually increased up to 24 hours a day, interrupted only for changing diapers.
- When the baby doesn't require intensive care, she ought to be transferred to the post-natal ward where KMC ought to be continued.

Can the mother continue KMC during sleep and resting?

A comfortable chair with adjustable back may be helpful to render KMC during sleep and rest. In the KMC ward or at home, the mother can sleep with the baby in kangaroo position in a reclined or semi-recumbent position, about 15 -30o degrees from above the ground. This can be attained with an adjustable bed, if available, or with several pillows on an ordinary bed.

It has bccn observed that this position may decrease the risk of apnea in a baby. A supporting garment to carry the baby in kangaroo position will allow the mother or the father or the relatives to sleep even with the baby in the kangaroo position. When the mother and the baby are well adapted to KMC they can be discharged from the hospital.

## FROM HOSPITAL TO HOME

### Criteria to Transfer the Baby from Nursery to the Ward

Standard criteria of the unit for transferring baby from the nursery to the post-natal ward ought to be as follows:

- Stable baby
- Gaining weight
- Mother confident to look after the baby

### Discharge Criteria

The standard policy of the unit for discharge from the hospital ought to be followed. In general the following criteria is accepted at most centres:

- Baby's normal health is good and no evidence of infections
- Feeding well, and receiving exclusively or predominantly breast milk.
- Gaining weight (at least 15-20 gm/kg/day for at least three consecutive days)
- Maintaining body temperature satisfactorily for at least three consecutive days in room temperature.
- The mother and family members are confident to take care of the baby in KMC and ought to be asked to come for follow-up visits on a regular basis.

When should KMC be discontinued ?

When the mother and baby are comfortable, KMC is continued for as long as possible, at the institution & then at home. Frequently this is desirable till the baby's gestation reaches term or the weight is around 2500 g. She starts wriggling to show that she is uncomfortable, pulls her limbs out, cries and fusses every time the mother tries to put her back skin to skin. This is the time to wean the baby from KMC. Mothers can render skin to skin contact occasionally after giving the baby a bath and during cold nights.

## POST-DISCHARGE FOLLOW UP

Close follow up is a fundamental pre-requisite of KMC practice. Though each unit should formulate its own policy of follow up. Generally, a baby is followed once or twice a week until 37-40 weeks of gestation or until the bay reaches 2.5-3 kg of weight. Smaller the baby at discharge, the earlier and more frequent follow-up visits should be. Thereafter, a follow up once in 2-4 weeks may be sufficient until 3 months of post-conceptional age. Later the baby ought to be seen at a gap of 1-2 months during first year of life. The baby should gain sufficient weight (15-20 gm/kg/day up to 40 weeks of post-conceptional age and 10 gm/kg/day subsequently). More frequent visits ought to be made if the baby is not growing well or his condition demands.

## NEONATAL UNIT

A neonatal intensive care unit, usually shortened NICU and also called a newborn intensive care unit, intensive care nursery (ICN), and special care baby unit (SCBU), is a unit of a hospital specializing in the care of ill or premature newborn infants. The NICU is distinct from the special care nursery (SCN) in providing a high level of intensive care to premature infants while the SCN provides specialized care for infants with less severe medical problems.

NICUs were developed in the 1950s and 1960s by paediatricians to provide better temperature support, isolation from infection risk, specialized feeding, and access to specialized equipment and resources. Infants are cared for in incubators or "open warmers." Some low birth weight infants need respiratory support ranging from extra oxygen (by head hood or nasal cannula) to continuous positive airway pressure (CPAP) or mechanical ventilation. Public access is limited, and staff and visitors are required to take precautions to reduce transmission of infection. Nearly all children's hospitals have NICUs, but they can be found in large general hospitals as well.

A NICU is typically directed by one or more neonatologists and staffed by nurses, nurse practitioners, Nursery Nurses, physician assistants, resident physicians, and respiratory therapists. Many other ancillary services are necessary for a top-level NICU. Other physicians, especially those with "organ-defined" specialties often assist in the care of these infants.

NICUs now concentrate on treating very small, premature, or otherwise sick babies. Some of these babies are from higher-order multiple births, but most are still single babies born too early. Premature labour, and how to prevent it, remain perplexing problems for doctors. Even though medical advancements allow doctors to save low birth weight babies, it is much better to be able to prevent it from happening in the first place.

Over the last 10 years or so, NICU have become much more 'parent friendly', encouraging maximum involvement with the babies. Routine gowns and masks have gone and parents are encouraged to help with care as much as possible. Cuddling, and skin-to-skin contact, also known as Kangaroo care, are seen as beneficial for all but the frailest (very tiny babies are exhausted by the stimulus of being handled, or larger critically ill infants). Less stressful ways of delivering high-technology medicine to tiny patients have been devised - stick-on sensors to measure blood oxygen levels through the skin, for example, and ways of reducing the amount of blood taken for tests.

Some major problems of the NICU have almost disappeared. Exchange transfusions, in which all the blood is removed and replaced, little by little, are rare now. Rhesus incompatibility (a difference in blood groups) between mother and baby is largely preventable. Breathing difficulties and brain haemorrhage still claims babies' lives and are the focus of many current research projects.

The long term outlook for premature babies saved by NICUs has always been a concern. From the early years, it was reported that a higher proportion than normal grew up with disabilities, including cerebral palsy and learning difficulties. Now that treatments are available for many of the problems faced by tiny or immature babies in the first weeks of life, long-term follow-up, and minimising long-term disability, are major research areas.

Besides prematurity and extreme low birth weight, common diseases cared for in a NICU include perinatal asphyxia, extreme cases of preeclampsia/eclampsia, major birth defects, sepsis, neonatal jaundice, and respiratory distress syndrome due to immaturity of the lungs. Complications of extreme prematurity may include intracranial haemorrhage, chronic bronchopulmonary dysplasia, or retinopathy of prematurity. An infant may spend a day of observation in a NICU or may spend many months there.

Neonatology and NICUs have greatly increased the survival of very low birth weight and extremely premature infants. In the era before NICUs, infants of birth weight less than 1400 grams (3 lb, usually about 30 weeks gestation) rarely survived. Today, infants of 500 grams at 26 weeks have a fair chance of survival.

The NICU environment provides challenges as well as benefits. Stressors for the infants can include continual light, a high level of noise, separation from their mothers, reduced physical contact, painful procedures, and interference with the opportunity to breastfeed. A NICU can be stressful for the staff as well. A special aspect of NICU stress for both parents and staff is that infants may survive, but with damage to the brain or eyes.

NICU rotations are essential aspects of paediatric and obstetric residency programs, but NICU experience is encouraged by other specialty residencies, such as family practice, surgery, Pharmacy, and emergency medicine.

## NICU IN INDIA

Neonatal mortality in India accounts for 50% of infant mortality, which has declined to 84/1000 live births. There is no prenatal care for over 50% of pregnant women, and over 80% deliver at home in unsafe and unsanitary conditions. Those women who do deliver in health facilities are unable to receive intensive neonatal care when essential. Level I and Level II neonatal care is unavailable in most health facilities in India, and in most developing countries. There is a need in India for Level III care units also. The establishment of neonatal intensive care units (NICUs) in India and developing countries would require space and location, finances, equipment, staff, protocols of care, and infection control measures. Neonatal mortality could be reduced by initially adding NICUs at a few key hospitals.

The recommendation is for 30 NICU beds per million population. Each bed would require 50 square feet per cradle and proper climate control. Funds would have to be diverted from adult care. The largest expenses would be in equipment purchase, maintenance, and repair. Trained technicians would be needed to operate and monitor the sophisticated ventilators and incubators. The nurse-patient ratio ought to be 1:1 and 1:2 for other infants. Training mothers to work in the NICUs would help ease the problems of trained nursing staff shortages. Protocols need not be highly technical; they could include the substitution of radiant warmers and room heaters for expensive incubators, the provision of breast milk, and the reduction of invasive procedures like venipuncture and intubation. Nosocomial infections ought to be reduced by vacuum cleaning and wet mopping with a disinfectant twice a day, changing disinfectants periodically, maintaining mops to avoid infections, decontamination of linen, daily changing of tubing, and cleaning and sterilizing oxygen hoods and resuscitation equipment, and maintaining an iatrogenic infection record book, which could be used to study the infection patterns and to apply the suitable antibiotics.

A neonatal intensive care unit is a unit that provides high quality skilled care to severely ill neonates by offering facilities for continuous clinical, biochemical and radiological monitoring and use of life support systems with the target of improving survival of these babies.

The notion of neonatal intensive care came into existence in the developed world in the mid-60's and 70's. With the availability of excellent maternal and child health services ensuing in survival of practically all normal newborns, their attention was then focussed on improving survival rates in the high risk group of newborns such as very low birth weight babies particularly those with problems such as hyaline membrane disease, babies with severe birth asphyxia, those with organ system failure leading to shock, coma, cardiac failure, babies with severe metabolic derangements or babies with major congenital malformations requiring surgery.

## STATUS OF NEONATAL CARE IN INDIA

Although the infant mortality rate (IMR) in our country has dropped from 144 per thousand live births to 84 per thousand five births in the past few decades, the neonatal mortality rate still accounts for over 50% of the IMR, What are the factors responsible for these demoralising figures? The deficiency starts with inadequate antenatal care. Over 50% of women have no access to basic antenatal care.

Over 80% of deliveries are still conducted at home with poor facilities for a safe and clean delivery by unskilled dais. Basic neonatal care (Level I) is not available at a majority of centres where neonates are delivered or admitted. Even larger hospitals with a high delivery rate do not have access to Level II neonatal care and the basic equipment required. Thus, a substantial decline in the neonatal mortality rate in our country can be achieved by improving components of neonatal care that don't require high levels of sophistication and technology. These include facilities for clean delivery and for resuscitation at birth, adequate temperature regulation, feeding of exclusive breast-milk, prevention of infection and early detection and prompt treatment of minor problems. Current emphasis therefore ought to be on improvement of Level I and if care so as to ensure survival of normal neonates and those with maximal chance for intact survival.

## NEED FOR NICUS IN INDIA

The question then arises whether neonatal intensive care units have a role in developing countries such as ours, taking into consideration the fact that neonatal intensive care is amongst the more expensive services that any healthcare system can render. Although enough data on the 'per patient' cost is not available in our country, in the USA the estimated average hospital cost of smallest surviving preterms exceeds US $ 1 lakh per year. Is it then justifiable to spend enormous sums of money to save a few babies when a majority of babies have no access to primary care?

The common cause of neonatal mortality in our country are asphyxia, prematurity and low birth weight, infections such as pneumonia and gastroenteritis and a variety of surgical problems. Although improved Level I and II care can bring down the mortality rates, simultaneous availability of good Level III care units are required for the large number of severely ill neonates that flood the few units where such facilities are available. Level III care areas consequently must be set up in those areas where Level II facilities have been operative successfully for quite some time. The setting up of such NICUs at apex institutions on a regional basis should run concurrently with programmes targeted at promoting Level I and II care in the society. According to present recommendations, about 30 NICU beds are recommended per million population.

The NICUs could be made responsible for training physicians and nurses working at Level II units and to assess and suggest modern technology in the Indian setting. Lastly, if family planning programmes in our country have to be effective, we ought to be able to ensure survival of the 'very sick neonates' which may only be possible with good intensive care.

## STATE-OF-THE-ART OF INTENSIVE CARE UNITS IN INDIA

Presently, there are only a few neonatal intensive care units in the country, majority of which are attached to teaching institutions. Over the past few years, a few privately run NICUs have mushroomed in some of the major cities. However, these are insufficient for the number of babies requiring intensive care and few babies can avail of these services due to the high costs. In spite of the fact that establishing and maintaining NICUs in a developing country are beset with a number of problems, the fact remains that there is a need for such units which ought to be developed in appropriate institutions on a regional basis.

## PROBLEMS ENCOUNTERED AND MODIFICATIONS REQUIRED

While setting up an NICU in a developing country, one has to face a number of problems and is bound down by many constraints. Very frequently, these problems can only be surmounted by making need based modifications as may be needed:

Space and location: The perfect method would be to allocate space for setting up NICU in the planning and constructions phase of an institution. This would ensure that the unit is suitably located near the delivery room and Obstetric OT to facilitate prompt transfer of babies. Also,, one can ensure that an average floor area of 50 square feet per cradle is available. Availability of some form of air handling units, air conditioners or a suitably placed exhaust fan is necessary for air exchange to occur in the unit without the occurrence of air draughts. Installation of the systems ought to be done at the inception of the intensive care unit. However, majority of NICUs in our country are not preplanned and consequently we may need to fit into the space made available.

Finances: The fundamental necessity for the development of any specialised care is the availability of enough finances. Unfortunately, in the distribution of finances in any given institution, the lion's share are diverted to adult care in ICCUs and MICUs with least preference for neonatal intensive care.

Equipment: A large part of the budget for an NICU is utilized for purchase of several types of equipment. Most of this equipment needs to be imported. Frequent breakdowns and poor maintenance and repair facilities result in a lot of equipment lying idle. Besides fundamental equipment for resuscitation, infusion, phototherapy and thermoregulation, a well equipped NICU needs a variety of sophisticated equipments such as cardiorespiratory, apnea monitors, blood pressure monitors, ventilators, infusion pumps, pulse oximeter and other equipment. However, the purchase of equipment ought to be in a phased manner and according to the need of the unit. Before finalizing a purchase, one should ensure that the equipment is sturdy, easy to clean, simple to operate user friendly and preferably indigenously manufactured. The company should have engineers offering prompt after sales service in the city, The availability of trained technicians and biomedical engineers in the hospital assists to prolong the life of the instrument.

Staff: The quality of services offered by an ICU depends not on the number of sophisticated incubators and ventilators but on the availability of clinical expertise round-the-clock, backed up by monitoring devices and equipment. Well-trained nurses and medical staff form the backbone of the service. Trained neonatal medical staff on call round-the-clock along with residents trained in neonatology for a minimum period of six months, are essential. In order to provide sufficient nursing care, the nurse-patient ratio ought to be 1:1 for babies on ventilator and 1:2 for all other babies, insufficient number of trained nursing staff, frequent transfers of existing staff coupled with overcrowding of NICU, interfere with the proper delivery of Level III care.

The shortage of nurses can be eased in part by encouraging entry of mothers into the NICU and involving them in the care of their baby. They can be entrusted with simple tasks such as changing their baby's diapers, assisting in feeding, even monitoring for colour and respiratory movements. No staff can be more dedicated than a mother helping to monitor her own baby's respiration, output or other parameters.

In addition, facilities for referral in the hospital to paediatric surgery, plastic surgery, cardiology and neurology are required.

Protocols of care: Although the term 'Intensive Care Unit' conjures the image of baby surrounded by a variety of beeping monitors and a mesh of wires, the term 'intensive care' need not be synonymous with ' invasive care'. In fact, the high incidence of nosocomial infections and iatrogenic problems necessitates that care in newborns be intensive in nursing skills but conservative in protocols of management'.

For instance, use of open care system of nursing under radiant warmers along with room heaters in winter in preference to incubators which are expensive, difficult to maintain and may be a source of infections. Avoiding use of parenteral fluids unless mandatory. Feeding all babies breastmilk by gavagelwati and spoon if unable to breastfeed and avoiding use of formula and bottles. Minimizing invasive procedures such as venelarterial punctures, intubation catheterisation, etc. are some of the measures found to be cost effective as they reduce need for higher antibiotics in addition to the cost of long hospital stay.

Infection control measures: Increased use of invasive interventions in severely ill neonates has made the hovering spectre of nosocomial infection a dreaded reality.

Prevention and control of nosocomial spread calls for a multi-disciplinary committee of administrator, microbiologist and clinicians, etc. of whom at least one of the persons in the committee supervises the day-to-day measures for infection control. These include:

Vacuum cleaning the area followed by wet mopping of the floors at least once every shift (thrice a day) with a disinfectant.

- Periodic changes in disinfectants to avoid resistant strains from emerging.

- Proper maintenance of mops which could otherwise be a source of organisms.
- Policy for decontamination of linen.
- Daily changing of suction and oxygen tubings, cleaning and sterilizing of oxygen hoods, resuscitation equipment.
- Maintaining an iatrogenic infection record book and the organisms; cultured, etc. so as to study the type of colonising organisms and to change usage of antibiotics as per the sensitivity pattern.

In conclusion, the high neonatal mortality rates pose a special problem in developing countries. The prompt need is to reduce these rates by making better Level I and II care for the neonates. In addition, neonatal intensive care ought to be developed concurrently at few apex institutions that serve as referral training and research centres.

## REFERENCES

Algranati PS. The pediatric patient: an approach to history and physical examination. Baltimore: Williams & Wilkins; 1992.

Algranati PS. Effect of developmental status on the approach to physical examination. Pediatr Clin North Am 1998; 45(1): 1-23.

Boynton R. Manual of ambulatory pediatrics, 4th edn. Philadelphia: Lippincott; 1998.

Brundige KJ. Preparing pediatric nurse practitioners for roles in specialty practice. J Pediatr Health Care 1997; 11(4):198-200.

Burns C. Pediatric primary care: a handbook for nurse practitioners, 2nd edn. London: WB Saunders; 2000.

Callender D. Pediatric practice guidelines: implications for nurse practitioners. J Pediatr Health Care 1999.

Engel J. Pocket guide to pediatric assessment, 3rd edn. St. Louis: Mosby; 1997.

Gaedeke MK. Advanced practice nursing in pediatric acute care. Crit Care Nurs Clin North Am 1995; 7(1):61-70.

Gill D, O'Brien N. Paediatric clinical examination, 3rd edn. London: Churchill Livingstone; 1998.

Jarvis C. Physical examination and health assessment, 2nd edn. Philadelphia: WB Saunders; 1996.

# 5

# Nursing Management in Common Childhood Diseases

## NUTRITIONAL DEFICIENCY DISORDERS

Malnutrition is a condition in which a person's diet is insufficient to meet minimum daily demands for nutrients like proteins, fats, vitamins, and minerals. It is caused by one of two factors. First, a person simply may not get sufficient food to eat and, thus, fails to take in the nutrients required to remain healthy.

Someone who is hungry all the time obviously is not eating sufficient food to remain healthy. Second, a person may eat a limited diet that fails to deliver vital nutrients to the body. Anyone who tries to survive on a diet consisting of potato chips, candy bars, and sodas will not be getting the comprehensive range of nutrients his or her body needs.

The single most significant factor that leads to malnourishment is poverty. Vast numbers of people who live in less-developed countries of the world either don't get sufficient to eat or don't eat the correct foods. Those who are most at risk of malnutrition where conditions of poverty exist are infants, children, pregnant women, and the senior.

Malnutrition is not restricted to less-developed nations, however. Even countries with high standards of living have their share of poor people who are underfed or poorly fed and may develop malnutrition. As per some estimates, at least 20 million Indians go hungry periodically within any given month.

All through the world, the death toll from malnutrition caused by hunger is estimated to range from 40,000 to 50,000 people a day. An additional 450 million to 1.3 billion people face the prospect of starvation from their limited food supplies.

Senior people in nursing homes or hospitals suffering from long-term illnesses or chronic metabolic disorders (which affect the way one's body processes food for energy) are also at risk for malnutrition. Health professionals have procedures to monitor the nutritional condition of these individuals. Malnutrition is also experienced by those suffering from a condition called anorexia nervosa, a disorder marked by a person's intentional refusal to eat correctly that can lead to starvation.

Nutrients serve a number of functions in the human body. Carbohydrates and fats, for instance, are used by the body to produce the energy humans require to stay alive and healthy and to grow and develop generally. Proteins are used in the production of new body parts, to protect the body against disease and infection, in the regulation of bodily functions, and in a variety of other ways.

Vitamins and minerals are used in the body for a number of different purposes, like controlling the rate at which many chemical changes take place in the body. Overall, more than 50 different nutrients are required to keep the human body healthy. The absence of any one of these nutrients can result in the development of a nutritional inadequacy disease. Some common nutritional deficiency diseases are discussed below.

## KWASHIORKOR AND MARASMUS

Kwashiorkor (from the West African word for "displaced child") is a nutritional deficiency disease caused when infants and very young children are weaned from their mother's milk and placed on a diet consisting of maize flour, cassava, or low-protein cereals.

That diet is in general high in calories and carbohydrates, but low in protein. The most striking symptom of kwashiorkor is oedema, a bloating caused by the accumulation of liquids under the skin. Other symptoms may include loss of hair and skin pigmentation, scaliness of the skin, and diarrhoea.

As the disease progresses, a person may develop anaemia (a disorder in which a person's red blood cell count is low and they lack energy), digestive disorders, brain damage, a loss of appetite, irritability, and apathy (lack of interest in things).

Most children don't die of kwashiorkor directly. Instead, they develop infections that, if left untreated, can be disastrous. They die from measles, the flu, diarrhoea, or other conditions that could be treated comparatively easily in a healthy child.

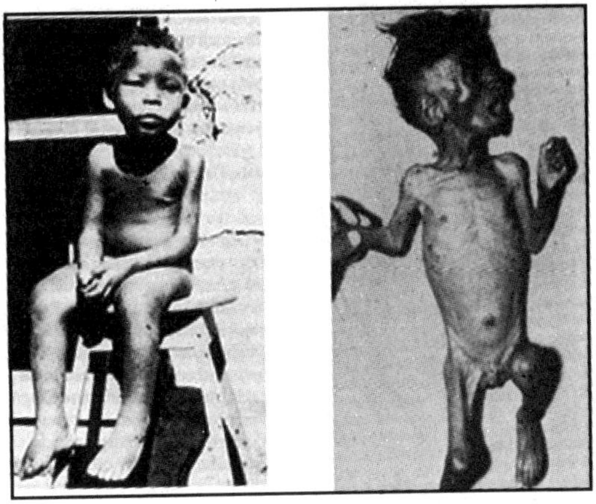


*Fig. Kwashiorkor and Marasmus*

Marasmus (from the Greek word for "to waste away") is a more severe condition than kwashiorkor. It results when a person's diet is low in both calories and protein. The disease is characterized by low body weight, wasting of muscle tissue, shrivelled skin, and diarrhoea. The most important feature of marasmus is a critically bloated belly. A child with marasmus has the appearance of an old person trapped in a young person's body.

## SCURVY

Scurvy is one of the oldest deficiency diseases recorded and the first one to be cured by adding a vitamin to the diet. It was a common disease amongst sailors during the age of exploration of the New World. Portuguese explorer Vasco da Gama (1460-1524) is said to have lost half his crew to scurvy in his journey around the Cape of Good Hope at the end of the fifteenth century.

The major symptom of scurvy is haemorrhaging, the heavy discharge of blood that results when a blood vessel is broken. The gums swell and usually become infected. Wounds heal slowly and the bleeding that occurs in or around vital organs can be disastrous. The disease is slow to develop and its early stages are characterized by fatigue (tiredness), irritability, and depression. In the advanced stages of the disease, laboratory tests will show an absence of the vitamin required to protect against the disease.

In 1747, a British naval doctor, James Lind (1716-1794), discovered the cause of scurvy. He found that sailors who were given oranges, lemons, and limes to eat along with their regular food did not develop scurvy. Despite this finding, it was not till the end of the eighteenth century that the British navy finally had its sailors drink a daily portion of lime or lemon juice to prevent scurvy.

The active ingredient in citrus fruits that prevents scurvy was not discovered till the 1930s. Then, two research teams, one headed by Hungarian-American biochemist Albert Szent-Györgyi (1893-1986) and the other by American biochemist Charles G. King, found that the antiscurvy agent in citrus fruits is a compound now known as vitamin C.

## BERIBERI

Beriberi is a disease that occurs widely in China, Indonesia, Malaysia, Burma, India, the Philippines, and other parts of Asia and the South Pacific Ocean. It is characterized by oedema (accumulation of water in body tissues), fatigue, loss of appetite, numbness or tingling in the legs, and normal weakness of the body. In fact, the name beriberi comes from the Singhalese word for "weakness."

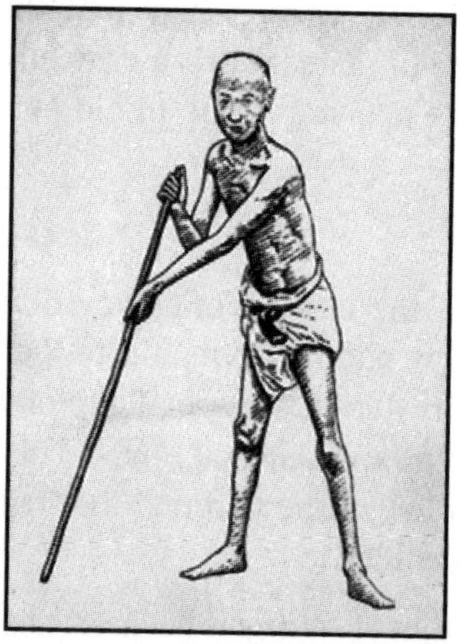

*Fig. Beriberi*

Beriberi is caused by an absence of vitamin B1 (thiamine) in the diet. The disease can be prevented by eating foods that are rich in this vitamin, foods like meats, wheat germ, whole grain and enriched bread, legumes (beans), peanuts, peanut butter, and nuts.

## PELLAGRA

The symptoms of pellagra are sometimes referred to as the "three Ds": diarrhoea, dermatitis, and dementia. Dermatitis refers to skin infections while dementia means deterioration of the mind. If the disease is not treated, it may lead to death. The cause for pellagra was discovered in the early twentieth century by Joseph Goldberger (1881-1929), a member of the United States Public Health Service. Goldberger established that pellagra is caused by an inadequate quantity of niacin (vitamin B3).

Niacin occurs naturally in foods like liver, meat, fish, legumes, and dried yeast. Today it is added to many processed foods like bread, flour, cornmeal, macaroni, and white rice. This practice has essentially eliminated pellagra as a medical problem in developed countries, though it remains a serious health problem in some less-developed countries of the world.

## RICKETS

Rickets is a bone disorder caused by a lack of vitamin D. Vitamin D is frequently called the "sunshine" vitamin because it can be produced in the human body by the effects of sunlight on the skin. Rickets was once a common disease of infants and children. However, all milk and infant formulas now have vitamin D added to them. Thus, the disorder is rarely seen today in countries where "fortified" milk is available. Symptoms of rickets include legs that have become bowed by the weight of the body and wrists and ankles that are thickened. Teeth may be badly affected and take a longer time to mature.

## OTHER VITAMIN DEFICIENCY DISEASES

The most common problem linked with a deficiency of vitamin A is night blindness. Night blindness is the inability to see well in the dark. Vitamin A is required for the formation of a pigment required by the eyes for night vision. Another eye disease caused by vitamin A deficiency is xerophthalmia, which can lead to blindness. This condition affects the cells of the cornea, other eye tissues, and the tear ducts, which stop secreting tears. Vitamin A deficiency is also responsible for a number of skin conditions, problems with tasting and smelling, and difficulties with the reproductive system.

Significant sources of vitamin A that can protect against such problems include fish-liver oils, butter, egg yolks, green and yellow vegetables, and milk. Vitamin E and K deficiencies are rare. A deficiency of vitamin E may be associated with sterility (inability to have children) and to more fast aging. Vitamin K promotes usual blood clotting.

Vitamin B12 (cobalamin) provides protection against pernicious anaemia and mental disorders. Vitamin B6 also protects against anaemia in addition to dermatitis, irritability, and convulsions.

## MINERAL DEFICIENCY DISEASES

About 25 mineral elements are needed in the human body for the maintenance of good health. Calcium and phosphorus, for instance, are required to produce teeth and bones. Diseases ensuing from the lack of a mineral are comparatively rare amongst humans. One of the exceptions is the disorder known as goitre. Goitre is a condition caused by an inadequate quantity of iodine in the diet. Iodine is used by the thyroid to produce hormones that control the body's usual functioning in addition to its usual growth. If enough iodine is not available in a person's diet, the thyroid gland begins to enlarge its cells in an effort to produce the required hormones. This enlargement produces the characteristic swelling in the neck characteristic of goitre. Today, goitre has virtually disappeared from most developed nations due to the practice of adding small quantities of iodine (in the form of sodium iodide) to ordinary table salt.

Perhaps the most common of all mineral deficiency disorders is anaemia. The term anaemia literally means "a lack of blood." The condition is caused when the number of red blood cells is reduced to a level lower than that essential for usual body functioning.

The human body gets the energy it needs to stay alive and function normally by oxidizing nutrients in cells. The oxygen required for this process is carried from the lungs to cells on red blood cells. The "working part" of a red blood cell is a complex molecule called haemoglobin. Each haemoglobin molecule contains a single atom of iron at its centre. The iron atom combines with oxygen from the lungs to form a compound known as oxyhaemoglobin. It is in this form that oxygen is transferred from the lungs to cells.

If the body fails to receive enough quantities of iron, a sufficient number of haemoglobin molecules will not be formed. In that case, there are not sufficient functioning red blood cells to carry all the oxygen that cells need to produce energy. A person becomes weak and listless and may suffer headaches, soreness of the mouth, drowsiness, slight fever, gastrointestinal disturbances, and other discomforts.

More than 30 different forms of anaemia have been recognized. These forms may result from a wide range of causes. For instance, a person who has surgery may lose sufficient blood to develop anaemia. A form of anaemia known as aplastic anaemia develops when bone marrow is destroyed by radiation, toxic chemicals, or certain types of medication. Loss of bone marrow arrests the production of red blood cells. haemolytic anaemia is caused by the rupture of red blood cells, a problem that can be caused by hereditary factors or by toxic agents.

## TREATMENT

The treatment for malnutrition and for nutrient deficiency diseases is obvious: a person who lacks sufficient quantities of food or fails to eat the right kinds of food must change his or her diet. That instruction is easy to give but in many parts of the world it is impossible to follow. Marasmus, kwashiorkor, beriberi, scurvy, rickets, and other deficiency disorders are common in less-developed countries of the world because enough food is either not available or, if it is, it is not adequately nutritious.

In more-developed countries of the world, people frequently have ready access to nutritious foods in enough quantities so that malnutrition is less of a problem than it is in less-developed countries. In addition, a very large variety of supplements are available, like vitamin and mineral pills. Anyone who fears that he or she may not be receiving enough of any given vitamin or mineral can easily supplement his or her diet with products available at the corner grocery store.

# RESPIRATORY DISORDERS AND INFECTIONS

The common cold, or acute nasopharyngitis, the most common respiratory disease in children, is caused by a large number of viruses and may be complicated by superimposed bacterial infection. There is no particular treatment.

Tonsillitis (acute infection of the tonsils) is more correctly believed to be a part of the acute-pharyngitis (throat-inflammation) syndrome. Enlargement of the tonsils as a result of recurrent infection frequently leads to the decision to remove the tonsils, a course many doctors now believe is rarely indicated. Enlarged tonsils don't cause irritability, poor appetite, or poor growth.

Enlargement of the adenoids (lymphoid tissue in the nasal part of the pharynx) as a result of recurrent infection can result in mouth breathing and a so-called adenoidal facial appearance, the most conspicuous feature of which is the constantly open mouth. By blocking the Eustachian tube, it can contribute to infections of the middle ear (otitis media) and to hearing loss. In children with chronic middle-ear disease and a particular type of hearing loss, removal of adenoids may be indicated.

Croup is an inflammatory disease of the larynx (voice box) or epiglottis (the plate of cartilage that shuts off the entrance into the larynx during the process of swallowing), most frequently caused by viral infection; it is encountered in infants and small children. Inflammation and swelling of the vocal cords lead to respiratory obstruction, especially in the inspiratory phase, and a croupy cough, which sounds such as the bark of a seal.

Allergic rhinitis (inflammation of the nasal passages) is the most common allergic disorder of childhood. Seasonal allergic rhinitis, or hay fever, because of sensitization to house dust, pollen, or molds, is characterized by attacks of sneezing, nasal itching, and a watery nasal discharge during the season when the particular allergens are prevalent. Similar symptoms are present in perennial allergic rhinitis but without seasonal pattern. In addition to inhalants, sensitization to particular foods may underlie the disorder. Treatment consists of avoidance of the substances causing the reaction, desensitization, and use of decongestant drugs and antihistamines (drugs that, by inactivating the histamine given off by injured cells, repress many of the symptoms of an allergic attack).

Asthma is a common allergic disorder of children that affects the bronchi and bronchioles (the large and small air passages in the lungs). Spasm, oedema, and abnormal secretion of mucus result in obstruction of the lower respiratory tract and characteristic wheezing and laboured breathing. Inhalant allergens, especially dust, molds, and pollens, and foods may play significant causal roles. Psychological stress may be a precipitating factor, but viral or bacterial infection of the respiratory tract is a more common triggering factor. A variety of effective treatments is available, together with preventive measures that reduce the chances of recurrent attacks. The outlook in general is good, with only a small percentage of children continuing to have severe asthma into adult life.

In discussing childhood respiratory diseases, tuberculosis and cystic fibrosis ought to be included. Both of these disorders predominantly affect the lungs, though many other organs may also be involved. Tuberculosis continues to be a major world health problem. As countries improve public-health standards and increase their socioeconomic level, the illness and mortality from this disease decrease steadily. Tuberculosis appears mostly in a primary form consisting of a small localized lesion of the lung that either heals completely or remains quiescent for many years. Only infrequently amongst children does the disease extend to involve other parts of the lung or other parts of the body, like bones, kidneys, or the central nervous system. Miliary tuberculosis, a generalized form of infection, and tuberculous meningitis are the most severe forms of the disease and have an extremely high mortality, though recuperation may occur with proper treatment. These forms most commonly occur in young children. As with other diseases, tuberculosis is better prevented than treated. A form of immunization (BCG-bacille Calmette-Guérin-vaccine) is utilized in areas of the world in which the disease is endemic. In other areas, control depends on prevention of contacts and early identification and treatment, if essential, of infected individuals. A variety of antibiotic agents is effective in treatment, especially the drugs isoniazid and rifampin.

Cystic fibrosis is a hereditary disorder of the exocrine glands (i.e., those glands that release secretions through ducts). It affects many organ systems, but the lungs suffer most critically. Estimates of incidence vary from one in 3,700 to one in 1,000 live births. It is rare amongst blacks and Orientals and is transmitted as a recessive trait. The underlying metabolic defect is unknown, but the disease appears to start with the secretion of unusually thick and sticky mucus. In foetuses, intestinal obstruction may result from the production of viscid meconium. Pulmonary involvement may be evident in the newborn or may develop during childhood, with repeated bouts of atelectasis (collapse of the lungs) and ultimate bronchiectasis (chronic dilation and degeneration of bronchi and bronchioles). Pancreatic insufficiency leads to a malabsorption syndrome, with fatty, bulky stools and malnutrition. The liver may be involved. Abnormality of the sweat glands is evidenced by a high salt content of the sweat, which, in hot weather, may lead to salt depletion and collapse. Treatment is directed toward the many organs involved, especially with regard to aggressive therapy for respiratory tract infections. Regulation of diet and administration of pancreatic enzymes contribute to the maintenance of sufficient nutrition. The ultimate outlook is grave, though therapy has been successful in noticeably prolonging life. Many affected persons survive into adult life.

Sinusitis, otitis, bronchitis (inflammation of the sinuses, the ears, and the bronchi, respectively), and pneumonia occur commonly in children and don't differ in necessary detail from the same diseases in adults. Other conditions that affect children and adults alike are described in respiratory disease.

## CONGENITAL DISORDERS

### CLEFT LIP AND PALATE

Cleft lip and palate are congenital anomalies ensuing in structural facial malformation. These defects are usually present in early foetal development. They are usually evident at birth and may be linked with any of more than 150 syndromes, with up to 13% of infants with cleft lip/palate having other birth defects.

The lip, or the lip and palate, fail to close in approximately one in every 1,000 neonates. Cleft lip (with or without cleft palate) occurs more often in males, and isolated cleft palate is more frequent in females. Cleft lip/palate is most prevalent amongst certain groups with the next most affected group being Asians (1.7 to 2.1 per 1,000 births), with Whites (1 per 1,000 births) and Blacks (0.3 per 1,000 births) following.

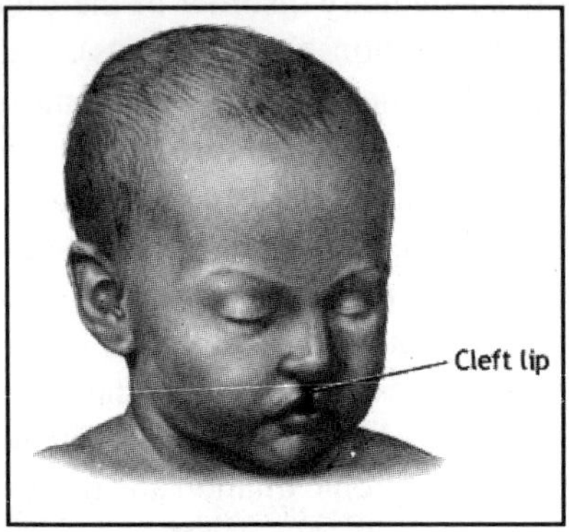


*Fig. Cleft Plate*

Combination of cleft lip and palate occurs in approximately 50% of cases; cleft lip alone occurs in about 25% of cases; and cleft palate alone occurs in about 25% of cases. The causes of oral clefts have been the subject of much study, but still remain poorly understood.

## Nursing Evaluation

- If the patient has a cleft lip, assess for cleft palate by direct visualization and palpation with finger.
- Obtain family history of cleft lip or palate.
- Evaluate feeding abilities.
  - Effectiveness of suck and swallow
  - Quantity taken
- Observe for other syndromic features.

## Nursing Diagnoses

- Ineffective Infant Feeding Pattern associated with defect
- Risk for Infection associated with open wound produced by malformation, ear infections

- Risk for Impaired Parent/Infant Attachment associated with malformation and special care needs
- Risk for Aspiration associated with tongue and palate deformities in Pierre Robin syndrome
- Deficient Knowledge associated with home management of infant with cleft malformation
- Fear associated with surgery
- Deficient Knowledge associated with postoperative care

## Nursing Interventions

Maintaining Adequate Nutrition:

- Administer gavage feedings if nipple feeding is to be delayed to prevent spread of a cleft lip.
- If sucking is permitted, use a soft nipple with crosscut to facilitate feeding. Note that nipples can be softened by boiling them.
- If sucking is ineffective because of inability to create a vacuum, try alternate oral feeding methods.
  - Feeding devices include preemie nipple, crosscut nipple, NUK nipple, Ross Cleft Palate Nurser, Haberman Feeder, or palatal obturator.
  - Avoid enlarging nipple holes because of infant's inability to control flow of milk, which will result in choking. Crosscut nipples allow milk to flow only when infant squeezes the crosscut open.
  - Using a squeezable bottle (e.g., Mead Johnson Cleft Palate Nurser) or plastic liner can be helpful by applying rhythmic pressure along with the infant's usual sucking and swallowing.
  - Rubber-tipped asepto syringe or dropper; the rubber extension ought to be long enough to extend back into the mouth to prevent regurgitation through the nose. Direct tip to side of mouth, and feed slowly.
- Feed infant in an upright, sitting position to decrease possibility of fluid being aspirated or returned through the nose or back to the auditory canal.
  - Feeding is usually easier if the nipple is angled to the side of the mouth away from the cleft so the infant's

tongue can press the nipple against the upper gum or dental arch.

- — Feed slowly over approximately 18 to 30 minutes. Feedings longer than 45 minutes expend too many calories and tire infant.
- — Smaller but more frequent feedings may be essential if the infant tires or requires extended time to eat.
- — Bubble regularly during feeding to decrease quantity of air swallowed.
- — Avoid repeated removal of nipple because of fear of choking. This may only frustrate the infant, causing crying and increasing chances of aspiration.
- — Feed infant before he or she becomes too hungry. If the infant is too agitated, feeding becomes a problem.

- Advance diet as suitable for age and requirements of infant. Eating usually improves when solids are introduced because they are easier for the infant to manipulate.
- Encourage the mother to start feeding the infant as soon as possible to enhance bonding and to strengthen the oral structures required later for mastication and speech production.
- Assist and support mother with breast-feeding if this is preferred.
  - — Suggest the use of a breast pump before nursing to stimulate the let-down reflex.
  - — Hold the infant in a semiupright, straddle, or football hold position.
- Nursing may need to be maintained and facilitated by using a breast pump and then bottle-feeding the pumped milk.

Preventing Infection:

- Protect child from infection so that surgery will not be delayed.
  - — Use and teach good hand-washing practice.
  - — Avoid patient contact with anyone who has an infection.
- Change the infant's position regularly.
- Clean the cleft after each feeding with water and a cotton-tipped applicator.
- Observe for fever, irritability, redness, or drainage around cleft, and report promptly.

- Monitor vital signs; report temperature greater than 101° F (38.3° C).

Promoting Acceptance and Adjustment:

- Show acceptance of the infant; maintain composure, and do not show negative emotion when handling the infant. The manner in which the nurse handles the infant can make a lasting impression on the parents.
- Support parents when showing a neonate for the first time. Demonstrate acceptance of the infant's and the parents' feelings. Parents may be grieving about the infant's cosmetic imperfections and may harbour ambivalent feelings about this infant.
- Offer information and answer any questions in a simple, matter-of-fact manner. The better informed the family, the easier it will be for them to see the infant as a normal child with a physical difference that will require surgery, dental work, and possibly speech therapy.
- Be aware that the usual sequence of parental responses may include shock, disbelief, worry, grief, and anger, and then proceed to a state of equilibrium and reorganization.
- Encourage parental involvement in infant's care: frequent holding, cuddling, and playing.

Preventing Aspiration and Airway Obstruction:

- When feeding the infant with Pierre Robin syndrome, consideration must be given to respiratory effort, flaccid tongue, and cleft palate. In general, feeding can be done with a nursing bottle (feeding techniques similar to those used for cleft palate).
  - — Use orthopneic position-vertical and slightly forward; this allows infant to push jaw forward to suck and allows the feeder a clear view of the infant.
  - — Use gentle finger pressure at mandibular attachment to bring the jaw forward.
  - — Feed slowly.
- Prevent respiratory obstruction by the tongue, particularly on inspiration and when the infant is quiet.
  - — Place the infant in prone position so tongue and jaw fall forward.

- — Tilt head back as tolerated by the infant, and slightly elevate upper trunk.
- — Place stockinette cap on infant's head and suspend from an overhead support to assist the infant to maintain a position for easy ventilation.
- — Suction nasopharynx as required.
- — If the tongue is sutured to pull it forward, observe for slipping, cut tongue, and infection.

- Observe closely for respiratory compromise.

Preparing for Home Management:

- Prepare family for home feedings by rendering several days to practice feeding and to become familiar with the infant's feeding pattern.
- Alert caregiver to difficulties with feeding and how to manage them.
    - — Nasal regurgitation: feed in more upright position or stop feeding and allow the infant a few seconds to cough or sneeze and clear the airway.
    - — Respiratory distress: feed slowly, and observe for aspiration.
    - — Longer feeding times: feed more often so infant does not tire.
- Suggest that about 1 week before scheduled admission for surgery the mother start using feeding techniques preferred by surgeon for postoperative feeding.
    - — Side of spoon
    - — Rubber-tipped dropper
    - — Toddler cup
- Encourage the parents to prepare siblings at home for the arrival of this infant. Suggest they show a picture of the new infant.
- Offer parents available literature about children with cleft lip and palate.
- Encourage parental involvement with local self-help groups that render information and parent-to-parent contact.
- Start referrals, as indicated, for extra support and financial assistance and early intervention programs.
- Describe and reinforce surgical treatment plans to the parents to promote communication and hope.

- Stress compliance with follow-up care with the paediatrician, plastic surgeon, dentist, orthodontist, psychologist, and speech therapist to prevent chronic otitis media, hearing loss, speech impairment, and emotional problems.
- Start a community nurse referral to continue emotional support and teaching progress at home.

## OESOPHAGEAL ATRESIA WITH TRACHEOESOPHAGEAL FISTULA

Oesophageal atresia (EA) is failure of the oesophagus to form a continuous passage from the pharynx to the stomach during embryonic development. Tracheoesophageal fistula (TEF) is an abnormal connection between the trachea and oesophagus. These disorders occur in 1 in 3,500 births, with a slight male dominance. Prematurity is common with oesophageal atresia or oesophageal atresia with a linked TEF, with 34% of these infants weighing less than 2,500 gm. Infants with pure TEF are in general not premature; their average gestational age is 37 weeks.

Approximately 50% of neonates with EA/TEF have other anomalies that vary in severity, with cardiac anomalies the most common (14.7% to 28%) and life-threatening. Linked anomalies include defects of the vertebrae, anorectal malformations, cardiac defects, renal defects, and defects of the radius or limbs.

### Nursing Evaluation

Evaluation begins promptly after birth.

- Be alert for risk factors of polyhydramnios and prematurity.
- Suspect in infant with the following:
  - Excessive quantity of mucus
  - Difficulty with secretions
  - Cyanotic episodes (unexplained)
- Report suspicion to healthcare provider promptly.

### Nursing Diagnoses

Preoperative:

- Risk for Aspiration associated with structural abnormality
- Risk for Deficient Fluid Volume associated with inability to take oral fluids
- Anxiety of parents associated with critical situation of neonate

Postoperative:

- Ineffective Airway Clearance associated with surgical intervention
- Ineffective Infant Feeding Pattern associated with defect
- Acute Pain associated with surgical procedure
- Impaired Tissue Integrity associated with postoperative drainage
- Risk for Injury associated with complex surgery
- Risk for Impaired Parent/Infant Attachment associated with prolonged hospitalization

## Nursing Interventions

### *Preoperative*

Preventing Aspiration:

- Position the infant with head and chest elevated 20 to 30 degrees to prevent or decrease reflux of gastric juices into the tracheobronchial tree.
  - This position may also ease respiratory effort by dropping the distended intestines away from the diaphragm.
  - Prone position will allow gastric juices to pool interiorly away from the oesophagus.
  - Turn often to prevent atelectasis and pneumonia.
- Perform intermittent nasopharyngeal suctioning or maintain indwelling Replogle tube (double-lumen tube) or sump tube with constant suction to remove secretions from oesophageal blind pouch.
  - Tip of tube is placed in the blind pouch.
  - Replogle or sump tube allows air to be drawn in through a second lumen and prevents tube obstruction by mucous membrane of pouch.
  - Maintain indwelling tube potency by irrigating with 1mL normal saline solution regularly.
  - Make sure that indwelling tube is changed as required and at least once every 12 to 24 hours (by the healthcare provider); alternate nostrils. Prevent necrosis of nostrils from pressure by catheter.

Place the infant in an Isolette or under a radiant warmer with high humidity to aid in liquefying secretions and thick mucus. Maintain the infant's temperature in thermoneutral zone, and ensure environmental isolation to prevent infection by using Isolette.

- Administer oxygen as required.
- Suction mouth to keep clear of secretions and prevent aspiration. Render mouth care.
- Be alert for indications of respiratory distress.
  - — Retractions
  - — Circumoral cyanosis
  - — Restlessness
  - — Nasal flaring
  - — Increased respiration and heart rate
- Maintain NPO status.
- Administer antibiotics as ordered to prevent or treat associated pneumonitis.
- Observe infant carefully for any change in condition; report changes promptly.
  - — Check vital signs, colour and quantity of secretions, abdominal distention, and respiratory distress.
  - — Evaluate for complications that can occur in any neonate or premature infant.
- Be available, and recognize need for emergency care or resuscitation.
  - — Have resuscitation equipment on hand.
  - — Accompany the infant to other departments and the operating room in Isolette with portable oxygen and suction equipment.
- Monitor for signs or symptoms that may indicate extra congenital anomalies or complications.
- Gastrostomy tube may be placed before definitive surgery to aid in gastric decompression and prevention of reflux. Maintain gastrostomy tube to straight gravity drainage, and do not irrigate before surgery.

Preventing Dehydration:

- Administer parenteral fluids and electrolytes as prescribed.
- Monitor vital signs regularly for changes in blood pressure (BP) and pulse, which may indicate dehydration or fluid volume overload.

- Record intake and output, including gastric drainage (if gastrostomy tube for decompression is present) and weight of diapers.

Reducing Parental Anxiety:

- Explain procedures and essential events to parents as soon as possible.
- Orient parents to hospital and intensive care nursery environment.
- Allow family to hold and assist in caring for infant.
- Offer reassurance and encouragement to family regularly. Render for extra support by social worker, clergy, and counsellor as required.

### Postoperative

Maintaining Patent Airway:

- Keep endotracheal (ET) tube patent by frequent lavage and suction. Note: Reintubation could damage the anastomosis.
- Suction regularly; every 5 to 10 minutes may be essential, but at least every 1 to 2 hours.
- Observe for signs of obstructed airway. Ventilatory support is continued till clinically stable (usually 24 to 48 hours)
- Request that the surgeon mark a suction catheter, indicating how far the catheter can be safely inserted without disturbing the anastomosis (usually ?¾ to 1 inch [2 to 3 cm]).
- Administer chest physiotherapy as prescribed.
  - Change the infant's position by turning; stimulate crying to promote full expansion of lungs.
  - Elevate head and shoulders 20 to 30 degrees.
  - Use mechanical vibrator 2 to 3 days postoperatively (to minimize trauma to anastomosis), followed by more vigorous physical therapy after the 3rd day.
  - Continue use of Isolette or radiant warmer with humidity.
  - Be prepared for an emergency: have emergency equipment available, including suction machine, catheter, oxygen, laryngoscope, ET tubes in varying sizes.

### Nursing Alert

Care ought to be taken not to hyperextend the neck, causing stress to the operative site.

Rendering Adequate Nutrition:

Feedings may be given by mouth, by gastrostomy, or (rarely) by a feeding tube into the oesophagus, depending upon the type of operation performed and the infant's condition. The gastrostomy is in general attached to gravity drainage for 3 days postoperatively, then elevated and left open to allow for air to escape and gastric secretions to pass into the duodenum before feedings are begun.

- Administer I.V. solutions until gastrostomy feedings can be commenced.
- Start gastrostomy feedings as soon as ordered because sufficient nutrition is a significant factor in healing.
  - Give the infant a pacifier to suck during feedings, unless contraindicated.
  - Use care to prevent air from entering the stomach, thereby causing gastric distention and possible reflux.
  - Continue gastrostomy feedings until the infant can tolerate full feedings orally.

Rendering Comfort Measures:

- Position comfortably.
- Avoid restraints when possible.
- Administer mouth care regularly.
- Offer pacifier regularly.
- Administer analgesics as ordered. Wean as soon as possible so ventilator can be discontinued without risk.
- Caress and speak or sing to infant regularly. Handling ought to be kept to a gentle minimum.

Maintaining Chest Drainage:

- Assess type of chest drainage present (determined by surgical approach). Report saliva or haemorrhage.
  - Retropleural-small tube in posterior mediastinum; may be left open for drainage
  - Transthoracic-chest tube placed in pleural space and connected to suction
- Keep tubing patent: free from clots, unkinked, and without tension.

- If a break occurs in the closed drainage system, immediately clamp tubing close to the infant to prevent pneumothorax.

Observing for Complications:

- Inspect for leak at the anastomosis, causing mediastinitis, pneumothorax, and saliva in chest tube: hypothermia or hyperthermia, severe respiratory distress, cyanosis, restlessness, weak pulses.
- Continue to monitor for complications during the recuperation process.
  - Stricture at the anastomosis: difficulty in swallowing, vomiting, or spitting up of ingested fluid; refusing to eat; fever secondary to aspiration and pneumonia
  - Recurrent fistula: coughing, choking, and cyanosis linked with feeding; excessive salivation; difficulty in swallowing linked with abnormal distention; repeated episodes of pneumonitis; normal poor physical condition (no weight gain)
  - Atelectasis or pneumonitis: aspiration, respiratory distress
- Render meticulous care for cervical esophagostomy-artificial opening in the neck that allows for drainage of the upper oesophagus.
  - Keep the area clean of saliva.
  - Wash with clear water.
  - Place an absorbent pad over the area.
- As soon as possible, allow the infant to suck a few ml. of milk at the same time gastrostomy feeding is being done. Advance the infant to solid foods as suitable if esophagostomy is maintained for a few months.
  - Encourage sucking and swallowing.
  - Familiarize the infant with food so that when able to eat orally, infant will be used to it.
- Start oral feedings 10 to 14 days postoperatively after anastomosis as directed.
  - Feed slowly to allow the infant time to swallow.
  - Use upright sitting position to avoid risk of regurgitation.
  - Bubble regularly.
  - Use demand feedings instead of strictly scheduled feedings.

— Do not allow the infant to become overtired at feeding time. Note cardiac rate.

— Try to make each feeding a pleasant experience for the infant. Use a consistent approach and patience. Encourage parental involvement.

Stimulating Parent-Infant Attachment:

- Gently hold and cuddle the infant for feedings and after feedings.
- Encourage parents to cuddle and talk to the infant.
- Render for visual, auditory, and tactile stimulation as suitable for the infant's physical condition and age.
- Render opportunities for the parents to learn all aspects of care of their infant.
- Encourage the parents to talk about their feelings, fears, and concerns.
- Help to develop a healthy parent-child relationship through flexible visiting, frequent phone calls, and encouraging physical contact between child and parents.

# CARDIOVASCULAR PROBLEMS

## CONGENITAL DEFECTS

As per a report, one in 125 babies born has a congenital (present at birth) heart defect - a problem that took place as the baby's heart was developing during pregnancy, before the baby is born. Congenital heart defects are the most common birth defects.

A baby's heart begins to develop at conception, but is completely formed by eight weeks into the pregnancy. Congenital heart defects happen during this vital first eight weeks of the baby's development. Particular steps must take place in order for the heart to form properly. Frequently, congenital heart defects are a result of one of these vital steps not happening at the right time, leaving a hole where a dividing wall should have formed, or a single blood vessel where two ought to be, for instance.

### Causes

The vast majority of congenital heart defects have no known cause. Mothers will frequently wonder if something they did during the pregnancy caused the heart problem. In most cases, nothing can be attributed to the heart defect. Some heart problems do occur more frequently in families, so there may be a genetic link to some heart defects. Some heart problems are likely to occur if the mother had a disease while pregnant and was taking medications, like anti-seizure medicines. However, most of the time, there is no identifiable reason as to why the heart defect occurred.

Congenital heart problems range from simple to complex. Some heart problems can be watched by the baby's doctor and managed with medicines, while others will require surgery, sometimes as soon as in the first few hours after birth. A baby may even "grow out" of some of the simpler heart problems, like patent ductus arteriosus (PDA) or atrial septal defect (ASD), because these defects may simply close up on their own with growth. Other babies will have a combination of defects and require several operations all through their lives.

## Different Types of Congenital Heart Defects

Chromosome Abnormalities and Congenital Heart Disease: Problems with chromosomes that result in genetic syndromes, like Down syndrome, frequently result in a higher incidence of infant heart malformations. Five to 8 percent of all babies with congenital heart disease have a chromosome abnormality. Chromosomes are the structures in the cells that contain the genes; genes code for the traits like eye colour and blood type. Usually there are 46 chromosomes in each cell of the body. Having too many or too few chromosomes results in health problems and birth defects. Structural defects of the chromosomes, where a piece of the chromosome is missing or present in duplicate, also causes health problems. There are a number of chromosome abnormalities linked with congenital heart defects. Some of these include the following:

- Down syndrome
- trisomy 18 and trisomy 13
- Turner's syndrome
- Cri du chat syndrome
- Wolf-Hirshhorn syndrome
- DiGeorge syndrome (deletion 22q11)

Chromosome analysis can be performed from a small blood sample to rule out the presence of a chromosome abnormality in a child with a congenital heart defect.

Single Gene Defects: There are an estimated 70,000 genes contained on the 46 chromosomes in each cell of the body. Genes come in pairs, one which is inherited from the mother, the other from the father. Genes not only compose our personal traits, but also compose health problems when gene alterations (mutations) are present. When a gene is mutated, a number of health problems may occur in a person, because of the single underlying genetic mutation. Several health problems with one genetic cause are frequently referred to as a syndrome. Some of the genetic syndromes linked with a higher incidence of heart defects include, but are not limited to, the following:

- Marfan syndrome
- Smith-Lemli-Opitz syndrome
- Ellis-van Creveld
- Holt-Oram syndrome
- Noonan syndrome
- Mucopolysaccharidoses

Other genetic syndromes which are not because of a single gene defect but are linked with congenital heart disease include Goldenhar syndrome (hemifacial microsomia), William's syndrome, and the VACTERL association (tracheal and oesophageal malformations linked with vertebral, anorectal, cardiac, renal, radial, and limb abnormalities make up the VACTERL syndrome).

When a child is born with a congenital heart defect, if there is a suspicion that the child has some type of genetic syndrome, a doctor who specializes in genetics (called a clinical geneticist) may be asked to assess the child.

If a child has been diagnosed with a chromosomal or other genetic abnormality, genetic counselling is useful to determine the risk of heart defects occurring in future children. Living with congenital (present at birth) heart disease calls for special care for the child.

## RHEUMATIC HEART DISEASE

Rheumatic heart disease is a condition in which permanent damage to heart valves is caused by rheumatic fever. The heart valve is damaged by a disease process that in general begins with a strep throat caused by bacteria called Streptococcus, and may eventually cause rheumatic fever.

Rheumatic fever is uncommon, except in children who have had strep infections that were untreated or inadequately treated. Children ages 5 to 15, especially if they experience frequent strep throat infections, are most at risk for developing rheumatic fever.

Rheumatic fever, an inflammatory disease, can affect many connective tissues, particularly in the heart, joints, skin, or brain. The infection frequently causes heart damage, especially scarring of the heart valves, forcing the heart to work harder to pump blood. The damage may resolve on its own, or it may be permanent, eventually causing congestive heart failure (a condition in which the heart can't pump out all of the blood that enters it, which leads to an accumulation of blood in the vessels leading to the heart and fluid in the body tissues).

## Symptoms

The symptoms of rheumatic fever usually begun about one to five weeks after the child has been infected with Streptococcus bacteria. The following are the most common symptoms of rheumatic fever. However, each child may experience symptoms differently. Symptoms may include:

- Joint inflammation - including swelling, tenderness, and redness over multiple joints. The joints affected are usually the larger joints in the knees or ankles. The inflammation "moves" from one joint to another over several days.
- Small nodules or hard, round bumps under the skin
- A change in the child's neuromuscular movements (this is usually noted by a change in the child's handwriting and may also include jerky movements)
- Rash (a pink rash with odd edges that is usually seen on the trunk of the body or arms and legs)
- Fever
- Weight loss
- Fatigue
- Stomach pains

The symptoms of rheumatic fever may resemble other conditions or medical problems. Always consult the child's doctor for a diagnosis.

## Treatment

Particular treatment for rheumatic heart disease will be determined by the child's doctor based on:

- The child's overall health and medical history
- Extent of the disease
- The child's tolerance for particular medications, procedures, or therapies

- Expectations for the course of the disease
- The opinion or preference

The best treatment for rheumatic heart disease is prevention. Antibiotics can usually treat strep throat (a Streptococcus bacterial infection) and stop acute rheumatic fever from developing. Antibiotic therapy has sharply reduced the incidence and mortality rate of rheumatic fever and rheumatic heart disease.

Children who have previously contracted rheumatic fever are frequently given continuous (daily or monthly) antibiotic treatments to prevent future attacks of rheumatic fever and lower the risk of heart damage.

If inflammation of the heart has developed, children may be placed on bed rest. Medications are given to reduce the inflammation, in addition to antibiotics to treat the Streptococcus infection. Other medications may be essential to handle congestive heart failure. If heart valve damage occurs, surgical repair or replacement of the valve may be considered.

# GENITOURINARY DISORDERS

## ACUTE GLOMERULONEPHRITIS

Acute glomerulonephritis is a broad term used to describe several disease processes that result in glomerular injury. The glomerular injury is the result of antigen-antibody deposits within the glomeruli. It occurs most often in school-age children, is rare in children younger than age 2, and occurs more often in males than in females (2:1).

### Nursing Evaluation

- Obtain history regarding recent streptococcal infection.
- Obtain suitable cultures and assess for present infection.
- Measure urine output and degree of haematuria and proteinuria.
- Weigh child and document areas and extent of oedema.
- Obtain baseline BP reading to assess for hypertension.

### Nursing Diagnoses

- Impaired Urinary Elimination associated with glomerular dysfunction
- Excess Fluid Volume associated with impaired renal function
- Deficient Diversional Activity associated with focus on fluid and salt restriction

- Deficient Knowledge regarding acute glomerulonephritis and its management

## Nursing Interventions

Promoting Normal Urine Output:

- Monitor daily intake and output.
- Test and record urine for haematuria and proteinuria as directed. Note colour of urine.
- Monitor daily weights.

Reducing Excess Fluid Volume:

- Render a no-added-salt diet during the acute phase of the illness. Other restrictions may be indicated if renal function is impaired. Protein intake is not usually restricted due to the possible risk of malnutrition.
- Restrict fluids in children with hypertension, oedema, heart failure, or renal failure.
- Place a sign that indicates dietary restrictions on the child's bed, so that staff and visitors will be aware of special requirements.
- With fluid restrictions, offer small quantities of fluids spaced at regular time interval all through the day and evening. Use a suitable size of cup for the quantity of fluid being offered.
- Check BP as ordered or required and observe for signs of hypertension. Administer antihypertensive drugs as ordered by healthcare provider.

Promoting Diversional Activity:

- Explain fluid restriction at an age-appropriate level and direct the child's focus away from restrictions.
- Render the child with diversional activity and play therapy.
- Encourage activity as tolerated.

Rendering Information:

- Explain all aspects of the diagnostic tests and treatment in terms the family can understand.
- Explain the purpose of all medications and the restricted diet, including a review of high-sodium foods to avoid and sample menus.

- Encourage family participation in the child's care.
- Help the family plan for adaptation of the child's nursing care to the home environment.
- Arrange for appointments for continued medical supervision and start referrals when appropriate.

## NEPHROTIC SYNDROME

Nephrotic syndrome is characterized by heavy proteinuria, hypoalbuminemia, and oedema. The syndrome can be subdivided into congenital, primary (idiopathic), and secondary types. Approximately 85% to 95% of primary cases in preadolescents are Minimal Change Nephrotic syndrome (MCNS) and are linked with minimal histologic change in the glomeruli. Nephrotic syndrome annually afflicts approximately 16 children per 100,000 younger than age 16; it is slightly more common in males than females in young children, but this disappears in teenagers and adults. Mean age at onset is 2½.

### Nursing Evaluation

- Obtain history of onset of illness and symptoms.
  - Precipitating events
  - Recent immunizations
  - Recent URIs
  - Flulike symptoms
  - Time of onset and location of oedema
  - Urinary pattern changes
- Perform physical examination focusing on vital signs; auscultation of breath sounds to determine adventitious sounds; areas and extent of oedema, particularly periorbital region, extremities, genitalia, abdomen; and peripheral perfusion, including pulses, colour, warmth of extremities.

### Nursing Diagnoses

- Excess Fluid Volume associated with fluid accumulation in tissues
- Risk for Infection associated with urinary loss of proteins and chronic steroid use
- Imbalanced Nutrition: Less Than Body Requirements associated with loss of proteins through urine and anorexia
- Interrupted Family Processes associated with childhood illness

## Nursing Interventions

Relieving Excess Fluid:

- Administer corticosteroids as suggested by the healthcare provider.
  - Observe for adverse effects and complications of therapy like Cushing's syndrome-increased body hair (hirsutism), rounding of the face ("moon face"), abdominal distention, striae, increased appetite with weight gain, cataracts, and aggravation of adolescent acne.
  - Stress that these physical changes are not unsafe or permanent and that they will disappear after the steroid treatment is stopped.
  - Observe for serious adverse effects and uncommon complications of corticosteroids.
- Administer immunosuppressive drugs as prescribed.
  - Make sure that patient and parents understand the desired and adverse effects of therapy.
  - Observe for complications of therapy, like decreased white blood cell (WBC) count, increased susceptibility to infection, hair loss or increased hair growth (hirsutism), gingival hyperplasia, haemorrhagic cystitis.
- Administer diuretics as prescribed.
  - Be aware of those diuretics that may cause potassium depletion.
  - Offer foods high in potassium, like orange juice, bananas, and dried fruits (e.g., raisins, apricots).
  - Administer supplemental potassium chloride as ordered and if the urine output is sufficient.
- Encourage activity as tolerated.
- Restrict fluids as ordered (usually only during the extreme edematous phases).
  - Restriction is carefully calculated at frequent time interval, based on the urine output of the previous day plus estimated insensible losses.
  - Offer small quantities of fluids spaced at regular time interval all through the day and evening. Use a cup of suitable size for the quantity of fluid being offered.

  - Measure fluids precisely in graduated containers. Don't estimate fluid intake or output.
  - Place a sign on the child's bed to make sure that no urine is accidentally discarded and that all intake is recorded.
  - Determine total intake and output every 8 hours. In children who are not toilet trained, a fairly accurate record of output can be obtained by weighing diapers before and after voiding.
  - Record other causes of fluid loss, like the number of stools per day, perspiration.
- Assist with abdominal paracentesis; this may be needed due to marked ascites. During the procedure, fluid is withdrawn from the peritoneal cavity to relieve pressure symptoms and respiratory distress.
- Restrict sodium as ordered (usually done while the child is proteinuric). A starting point is 2 to 3 g/day.
  - Use a low-sodium menu when ordering meals from the hospital.
  - Assist family in making food choices that are low in sodium.
  - Foods that ought to be limited include cured, salted, canned, or smoked meats; processed cheese; regular canned or frozen soups and bouillon cubes; salted crackers and other snack foods.

### Nursing Alert

No live vaccinations or immunizations ought to be given during active episodes of nephrosis or while the child receives immunosuppressive therapy.

## TUMORS OF THE KIDNEY

Renal tumors in the newborn infant are uncommon and include congenital mesoblastic nephroma, multilocular cystic nephroma, and Wilms tumor (i.e., nephroblastoma). Other renal neoplasms, including renal cell carcinoma, rhabdoid tumor, lymphoma, and teratoma, are rare in the newborn infant. The clinical presentation of a renal tumor in the neonatal period is usually that of abdominal swelling or a palpable mass. There may be hypertension, haematuria, fever, and feeding intolerance.

Congenital mesoblastic nephroma is the most common renal neoplasm in the first year of life. Approximately 60% of all congenital mesoblastic nephromas are diagnosed before 6 months of age; the clinical presentation is an abdominal mass. Congestive heart failure and hypertension are less common manifestations. Nephrectomy is curative, with the exception of infrequent local recurrences and rare pulmonary metastases.

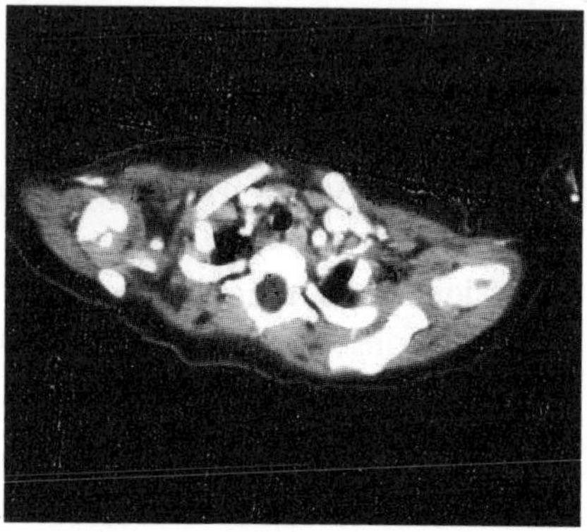

*Fig. Tumors of the Kidney*

Multilocular cystic nephroma is a benign renal tumor that consists of large cysts separated by fibrous septa. This tumor arises from metanephric blastema and has features of immature blastema, tubules, and skeletal muscle on histopathologic examination. The prognosis is excellent with surgical removal alone for these patients.

Wilms tumor is a malignancy that accounts for 90% of all renal tumors diagnosed in the pediatric population. However, 80% of all Wilms tumors are diagnosed in patients between the ages of 1 and 5 years, making its appearance uncommon in the first year of life and rare in the first month of life.

Most of these tumors occur sporadically, but 15% are associated with congenital anomalies or syndromes, including congenital aniridia, hemihypertrophy, WAGR syndrome (i.e., Wilms tumor, aniridia, genitourinary anomalies, and mental retardation), Denys-Drash syndrome (i.e., Wilms tumor, male pseudohermaphroditism, and nephrotic syndrome caused by diffuse mesangial sclerosis), and Beckwith-Wiedemann syndrome (i.e., omphalocele, macroglossia, and visceromegaly). Two candidate genes for Wilms tumor have been localized: its suppressor gene WT1, which is located on chromosome 11p13, and another gene on chromosome 11p15.

Definitive therapy for a localized renal mass begins with surgical exploration, and in most cases the primary treatment is nephrectomy. Infants with multilocular cystic nephromas or congenital mesoblastic nephromas require no postoperative therapy. Infants with malignant tumors such as Wilms tumor are treated according to well established oncologic protocols. The prognosis for most infants with neonatal renal tumors is good, although an infant with an aggressive Wilms tumor, an atypical congenital mesoblastic nephroma, or a renal sarcoma may have a poor prognosis.

## NEUROLOGIC INFECTIONS AND DISORDERS

## CEREBRAL PALSY

Cerebral palsy is a complete diagnostic term used to designate a group of nonprogressive disorders ensuing from malfunction of the motor centres and pathways of the brain. Though there are varying degrees and clinical manifestations of cerebral palsy, it is in general characterized by paralysis, weakness, incoordination, or ataxia. Cerebral palsy occurs in approximately 2 per 1,000 live births. It is a major cause of disability amongst children.

### Nursing Evaluation

- Perform a functional evaluation; determine ability to perform activities of daily living (ADLs).
- Perform a developmental evaluation; use Denver II developmental or other screening tool.
- Evaluate ability to protect airway-gag reflex, swallowing.
- Assess nutritional status-growth, signs of deficiency.
- Assess neuromuscular function and mobility-range of motion (ROM), spasticity, coordination.
- Assess speech, hearing, vision.
- Evaluate parent-child interactions.
- Determine parents' understanding of and compliance with treatment plan.

### Nursing Diagnoses

- Impaired Physical Mobility associated with altered neuromuscular functioning

- Delayed Development and growth associated with the nature and extent of the disorder
- Interrupted Family Processes associated with the nature of the defect, the requirements of daily management, and resultant changes in family life
- Risk for Injury associated with deficit in motor activity and coordination

## Nursing Interventions

Increasing Mobility and Minimizing Deformity:

- Carry out and teach the parents to carry out suitable exercises under the direction of the physical therapist.
- Use splints and braces to facilitate muscle control and improve body functioning.
  - Apply as directed.
  - Remove for suggested time.
  - Inspect underlying skin for redness and irritation, signs of improper application, or poor fit.
- Use assistive devices, like adapted grooming tools, writing implements, and utensils, to enhance independence. Handles of toothbrushes, spoons, and forks can be built up with sponges or specifically curved to make holding easier.
- Encourage self-dressing with easy pull-on pants, large sweatshirts, Velcro closures, and other loose clothing.
- Use play, like board games, ball games, pegboards, and puzzles, to improve coordination.
- Maintain good body alignment to prevent contractures.
- Render sufficient rest periods.
  - Avoid exciting events before rest or bedtime.
  - Administer or teach parents to administer muscle relaxants or anticonvulsants as prescribed.
  - Schedule physical therapy after child has rested, and avoid stress and frustration during physical therapy.

## HYDROCEPHALUS

Hydrocephalus is a condition of altered production, flow, or absorption of cerebrospinal fluid (CSF). It is characterized by an abnormal increase in CSF volume within the intracranial cavity and by enlargement f the head in infancy. Occurs in approximately three to four cases per ,000 births, including those linked with spina bifida.

## lursing Evaluation

- Assess head circumference.
  - Measure at the occipitofrontal circumference-point of largest measurement.
  - Measure the head at approximately the same time each day.
  - Use a centimeter measure for greatest accuracy.
- Palpate fontanelle for tenseness, bulging.
- Assess pupillary response.
- Assess level of consciousness (LOC).
- Evaluate breathing patterns and effectiveness.
- Assess feeding patterns and patterns of emesis.
- Assess motor function, gait, coordination.
- Determine attainment of developmental milestones.

## lursing Diagnoses

- Ineffective Cerebral Tissue Perfusion associated with increased ICP before surgery
- Imbalanced Nutrition: Less Than Body Requirements associated with reduced oral intake and vomiting
- Risk for Impaired Skin Integrity associated with alterations in LOC and enlarged head
- Anxiety of parents associated with child undergoing surgery
- Risk for Injury associated with malfunctioning shunt
- Risk for Deficient Fluid Volume associated with CSF drainage, decreased intake postoperatively
- Risk for Infection associated with bacterial infiltration of the shunt
- Ineffective Family Coping associated with diagnosis and surgery

## Nursing Interventions

- Observe for evidence of increased ICP, and report promptly.
- Assist with diagnostic procedures to determine cause of hydrocephalus and indication for surgical intervention.

— Explain the procedure to the child and parents at the levels of comprehension.
— Administer prescribed sedatives half hour before th procedure to ensure their effectiveness.
— Organize activities so the child is permitted to rest aft administration of the sedative.
— Observe closely after ventriculography for the following

- Leaking of CSF from the sites of subdural or ventricular tap These tap holes ought to be covered with a small piece o gauze or cotton saturated with collodion.
- Reactions to the sedative, particularly respiratory depression.
- Changes in vital signs indicative of shock.
- Signs of increased ICP, which may occur if air has been injecte into the ventricles.

## SPINA BIFIDA

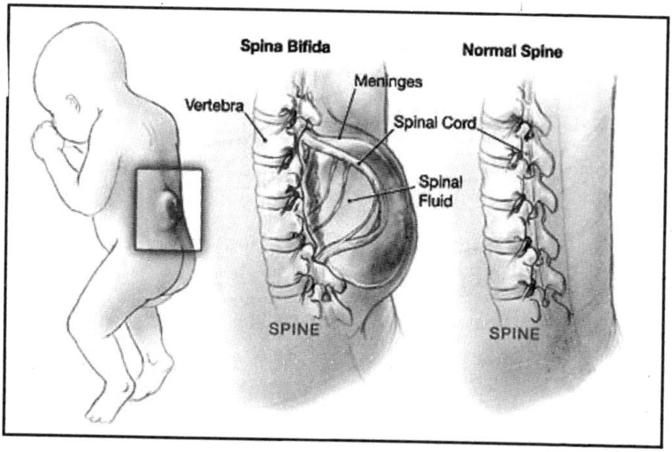


*Fig. Spina Bifida*

Spina bifida, also called spinal dysraphia, is a malformation of the spine in which the posterior portion of the laminae of the vertebrae fails to close. It occurs in approximately 1 per 1,000 live births and is the most common developmental defect of the central nervous system (CNS). Several types of spina bifida are recognized, of which the following three are most common.

### Spina Bifida Occulta

- The defect is only in the vertebrae. The spinal cord and meninges are normal.

- Meningocele
- The meninges protrude through the opening in the spinal canal. This forms a cyst filled with CSF and covered with skin.
- Myelomeningocele (or Meningomyelocele)
- The spinal cord and cord membranes protrude through the defect in the laminae of the vertebral column. Myelomeningoceles are covered by a thin membrane.

## ursing Evaluation

- Assess sensory and motor response of lower extremities.
- Assess ability to void spontaneously, retention of urine, symptoms of UTI.
- Assess usual stooling patterns, need for medications to facilitate elimination.
- Assess mobility and use of braces, casts, and other special equipment.

## ursing Diagnoses

- Risk for Impaired Skin Integrity associated with impaired motor and sensory function
- Risk for Infection associated with contamination of the myelomeningocele site
- Impaired Urinary Elimination associated with neurologic deficits
- Ineffective Tissue Perfusion: Cerebral associated with potential hydrocephalus
- Fear (parents) associated with neonate with neurologic disorder and to surgery
- Ineffective Thermoregulation following surgery
- Impaired Urinary Elimination associated with sacral denervation
- Bowel Incontinence or Constipation associated with impaired innervation of anal sphincter and bowel musculature
- Disturbed Body Image associated with the child's appearance, difficulties with locomotion, and lack of control over excretory functions

## ursing Interventions

- Avoid positioning on the infant's back to prevent pressure on the sac. Check position at least once every hour.

- Don't place a diaper or other covering directly over the sac.
- Observe the sac regularly for evidence of irritation or leakag of CSF.
- Use prone positioning with hips only slightly flexed to decreas tension on the sac.
- Place a foam rubber pad covered with a soft cloth betwee the infant's legs to maintain the hips in abduction and to preve or counteract subluxation. A diaper roll or small pillow may b used in place of the foam rubber pad.
- Allow the infant's feet to hang freely over the pads or mattres edge to prevent aggravation of foot deformities.
- Render meticulous skin care to all areas of the body, particularl ankles, knees, tip of nose, cheeks, and chin.
- Render passive ROM exercises for muscles and joints that th infant doesn't use spontaneously. Avoid hip exercises due t common hip dislocation, unless otherwise suggested.
- Use a foam or fleece pad to reduce pressure of the mattres against the infant's skin.
- Avoid pressure on the infant's back during feeding by holdin the infant with the elbow rotated to avoid touching the sac, o feeding while infant is lying on side or prone on the lap Encourage the parents to use these positions to render infan stimulation and bonding.

## MENINGITIS

Bacterial meningitis is an inflammation of the meninges that follow the invasion of the spinal fluid by a bacterial agent. Most cases are seen i children younger than age 5.

### Nursing Evaluation

- Obtain a history from the parents about recent upper respirator or other infection.
- Assess LOC and neurologic status.
  - — Evaluate for Kernig's sign-with the child in the supin position and knees flexed, flex the leg at the hip so th thigh is brought to a position perpendicular to the trunk Attempt to extend the knee. If meningeal irritation i present, this can't be done, and attempts to extend th knee result in pain.

— Evaluate for Brudzinski's sign-flex the patient's neck. Spontaneous flexion of the lower extremities indicates meningeal irritation.

- Monitor breathing pattern and circulatory status.

## Nursing Diagnoses

- Ineffective Tissue Perfusion: Cerebral associated with endotoxin release into the CSF
- Hyperthermia associated with infectious process
- Acute Pain associated with neurologic effects from the disease process
- Risk for Infection transmission associated with bacterial agents
- Ineffective Tissue Perfusion: Cerebral associated with complications of infectious process
- Anxiety of parents associated with severity of illness and hospitalization

## Nursing Interventions

- Administer antimicrobial agents at specified time intervals to obtain optimal serum levels. Obtain blood studies for peak and trough levels as ordered.
- Maintain patent I.V. line for medication administration; observe for signs of infiltration and phlebitis.
- Monitor closely for signs of complications affecting cerebral perfusion.
  — Monitor vital signs, LOC, and neurologic status at frequent time interval.
  — Monitor intake and output, weight, and head circumference daily to assess for hydrocephalus.
  — Be particularly alert for lethargy or subtle changes in condition, which may indicate cerebral oedema.
  — Precisely chart child's behaviour and clinical signs.
- Administer antipyretics, tepid sponge baths, and hypothermia blanket as ordered to reduce fever. Fever increases metabolic rate and energy demands by the brain; this may lead to hypoxemia and brain damage in the child with cerebral vascular compromise.
- Monitor for seizures and use seizure precautions in the febrile child.

  - There is an increased potential for seizures in the febrile child.
  - Ensure safety by using padded bed or crib rails and having airway and suction equipment on hand.
- Reduce the normal noise level around the child, and prevent sudden loud noises.
- Organize nursing care to render for periods of uninterrupted rest.
- Keep normal handling of the child at a minimum. When essential, approach the child slowly and gently.
- Maintain subdued lighting as much as possible.
- Speak in a low, well-modulated tone of voice.
- Medicate for pain as ordered, avoiding opioids that cause CNS and respiratory depression.

## EPILEPSY

Seizure disorder is a term used to encompass a number of varieties of episodic disturbances of brain function. Seizures shouldn't be considered as one particular disease, but as a symptom of an underlying disorder. They are rather common in children, being more prevalent during the first 2 years than at any other time in life. Incidence of epilepsy is estimated at 15 cases per 100,000 population. Of individuals with seizure disorders, 90% are diagnosed before age 20.

### Nursing Evaluation

- During a seizure, assess the following:
  - Indications of difficulties with airway or breathing.
  - Significant preseizure events, like noise, excitement, lethargy.
  - Behavior before the seizure, aura.
  - Types of movements observed.
  - Time seizure started and ended.
  - Site where twitching or contraction started.
  - Areas of the body involved.
  - Movements of the eyes and changes in pupil size.
  - Incontinence.
  - Colour change-pallor, cyanosis, flushing.
  - Mouth-teeth clenched, abnormal movements, tongue bitten.
  - Apparent degree of consciousness during the seizure.

- After a seizure, assess the following:
  - — Degree of memory for recent events.
  - — Types of speech.
  - — Coordination, paralysis, or weakness.
  - — Length of time the child is postictal.
  - — Pupillary reaction.
  - — Vital signs.

## Nursing Diagnoses

- Risk for Injury associated with seizure activity
- Ineffective Breathing Pattern associated with spasms of respiratory musculature
- Social Isolation associated with the child's feelings about seizures or public fears and misconceptions
- Chronic Low Self-Esteem associated with lack of control over seizures

## Nursing Interventions

- Use preventive measures.
  - — Remove hard toys from the bed.
  - — Pad the sides of the crib or side rails of the bed.
  - — Have a suction machine available to remove secretions during a seizure.
  - — Have an emergency oxygen source in the room in case of sudden respiratory difficulty.
- Make sure the child can be readily observed.
- During a seizure, monitor vital signs and assess neurologic status regularly.
- After a seizure, check the child regularly and report the following:
  - — Behavior changes.
  - — Irritability.
  - — Restlessness.
  - — Listlessness.
- During a seizure, take the following emergency actions:
  - — Clear the area around the child.
  - — Don't restrain the child.

- — Loosen the clothing around the neck.
- — Turn the child on side so saliva can flow out of the mouth.
- — Place a small, folded blanket under the head to prevent trauma if the seizure occurs when the child is on the floor.

- Suction the child, and administer oxygen as essential.
- Don't give anything by mouth or attempt to place anything in the mouth.
- After the seizure, place the child in a side-lying position.

## HAEMATOLOGIC DISORDERS

### ANAEMIA

Anaemia refers to a deficit of red blood cells (RBC) or haemoglobin (Hb) in the blood, ensuing in decreased oxygen-carrying capacity. It is the most frequent haematologic disorder encountered in children.

### Nursing Evaluation

- Obtain history of potential causes.
  - — Dietary history, including the quantity of milk and meat consumed; medications.
  - — Family history for genetic causes.
  - — Persistent infection, fever, or chronic disease.
  - — Exposure to drugs, poisons.
  - — Pica-craving and consuming nonfood items (e.g., paint chips, ice, paper).
- Obtain a baseline evaluation.
  - — Observe skin and mucous membranes for pallor.
  - — Obtain height and weight and plot on growth curve.
  - — Measure vital signs, including blood pressure (BP).
  - — Assess child's functional level-level of exercise tolerance, mental functioning.
  - — Assess attainment of developmental milestones.
- Observe for fatigue, listlessness, irritability.
- Observe for blood loss: bruising, bleeding, haematuria, or haematochezia (blood in stool). Assess for excessive menstrual bleeding in adolescent females.

## Nursing Alert

Be alert for children at risk for iron deficiency anaemia-children in fast growth stages (toddlers and adolescents) and pregnant or lactating adolescents.

## Nursing Diagnoses

- Fatigue associated with decreased ability of blood to transport oxygen to the tissues
- Imbalanced Nutrition: Less Than Body Requirements of suggested daily dietary allowances
- Risk for Infection associated with debilitated state
- Anxiety associated with hospitalization and painful diagnostic procedures (venipunctures, finger sticks)
- Delayed Development and growth associated with decreased energy

## Nursing Interventions

Minimizing Fatigue:

- Plan nursing care to allow for lengthy periods when the child is not disturbed by hospital routines, procedures, treatments; set priorities.
- Observe for early signs of fatigue, like irritability, hyperactivity, listless.
- Encourage sedentary instead of active projects.
- Administer oxygen and position upright if dyspnoea present.
- Don't always encourage self-care.
- Render finger foods that are easy to chew to conserve energy.

Rendering Adequate Nutritional Intake:

- Be aware of the child's food preferences and plan diet accordingly.
- Offer small quantities of food at frequent time interval.
- Reward the child for positive attempts to eat.
- Allow the child to participate in selection of foods and in preparation of meal tray.
- Avoid tiring activities and unpleasant procedures at mealtime.
- Make mealtime as pleasurable as possible.

- Render iron-rich food and vitamins when essential.
- If iron is ordered, give between meals and with orange juice (iron is absorbed best in an acidic environment).
- Limit milk and milk products to 16 oz to 24 oz per day. Milk products arrest the absorption of oral iron.
- Administer liquid iron with a dropper or straw or dilute with water or fruit juice to prevent staining of the teeth.
  - — If given by dropper, make sure that liquid iron is deposited in the back of the mouth.
  - — Dental stains can be removed by brushing the teeth with sodium bicarbonate or hydrogen peroxide and then rinsing with water after each administration.
- Be alert for adverse effects of iron supplements-gastric distress, colic pain, diarrhea, or constipation; may call for decreased dose.
- Advise family that child's stool may turn dark green or black.
- Stress the importance of continuing iron therapy as per healthcare provider's directions, although the child may not appear to be ill.
- Inform parents that iron overdoses can be unsafe or disastrous.

## THALASSEMIA

Thalassemia major is the most severe of the beta-thalassemia syndromes and represents the homozygous form of the disease. Beta-thalassemia (thalassemia) refers to an inherited haemolytic anaemia, characterized by a reduction or absence of the globulin chain in Hbsynthesis. This RBC has a decreased quantity of Hb, ensuing in a fragile RBC with a short life span. Most prevalent in the Mediterranean basin, Middle East, Southeast Asia, and Africa. It is most common in children of Italian, Greek, and Southeastern Asian ancestry.

### Nursing Evaluation

- Obtain family history of thalassemia or unexplained anaemia or heart failure.
- Perform whole body examination to assess for anaemia and systemic complications of thalassemia.
- Measure development and growth parameters.

## Nursing Diagnoses

- Ineffective Tissue Perfusion associated with abnormal Hb
- Chronic Pain associated with progression of disease in bone
- Activity Intolerance associated with bone pain, cardiac dysfunction, and anaemia
- Risk for Infection associated with progressive anaemia and splenectomy
- Deficient Knowledge associated with iron chelation therapy
- Disturbed Body Image associated with endocrine and skeletal abnormalities
- Ineffective Family Coping associated with poor prognosis

## Nursing Interventions

Maximizing Tissue Perfusion:

- Administer blood transfusions as ordered.
  - Observe for signs of transfusion reaction (increased chance caused by frequency) including allergic, febrile, septic, circulatory overload, and haemolytic reactions.
  - Allergic reactions usually occur within 15 to 20 minutes of start of the transfusion, though delayed reactions may occur up to several months later.
- Monitor cardiovascular status for complications.
  - Monitor apical pulse, BP, and respirations.
  - Assess for oedema.
  - Auscultate heart sounds for gallop and lungs for rales.
  - Assess extremities for ulcer formation.
- Refer to care of the child with heart failure.

Relieving Bone Pain:

- Monitor CBC as ordered and report Hb levels of less than 10 g/dL.
- Elevate lower extremities.
- Render warm baths or soaks.
- Administer or teach proper administration of NSAIDs, like ibuprofen (Motrin) or naproxen (Naprosyn). Use carefully and monitor liver enzymes in patients with liver complications.

Minimizing Activity Intolerance:

- Encourage participation in activities that don't require significant strenuous activity. Full participation in some activities, particularly with peers, will increase self-esteem.
- Facilitate physical and occupational therapy consultation to develop an acceptable exercise plan.
- Assist the parents in contacting the child's school and develop a plan of gym activities, classes, and rest periods that allow the greatest level of participation and slowly develop endurance. Advise parents that during the week of the scheduled transfusion, the fatigue will be greatest, so gym and other exertional activities ought to be modified.
- Suggest that driving the child to school and rendering sufficient rest at home will render her with more energy for school activities.
- Discourage participation in contact or other sports that increase the child's risk for a fracture (skateboarding, football, soccer).

## HAEMOPHILIA

Haemophilia is usually an inherited, congenital bleeding disorder characterized by a lack of blood clotting factors, particularly factors VIII and IX. It is an X-linked disorder primarily affecting males; females act as carriers. Occurs in 1 in 5,000 males. There is no racial predilection, and haemophilia is found in all ethnic groups.

- 80% to 85% have factor VIII deficiency or haemophilia A (classic haemophilia).
- 15% to 20% have factor IX deficiency or haemophilia B (Christmas disease).
- Few have factor XI deficiency or haemophilia C.

### Nursing Evaluation

- Obtain history of and observe for unusual bleeding-ecchymosis, prolonged bleeding from mucous membranes and lacerations, haematomas, haemarthroses, haematuria, rectal and GI bleeding.
- Assess joints for swelling, warmth, tenderness, range of motion (ROM), contractures, and surrounding muscle atrophy.
- Assess family resources and coping skills.

## Nursing Diagnoses

- Risk for Deficient Fluid Volume associated with haemorrhage.
- Ineffective Protection associated with inability of blood to clot.
- Impaired Physical Mobility associated with repeated haemarthroses.
- Acute Pain associated with bleeding into joints and muscles.
- Ineffective Family Coping associated with disabling and life-threatening disease.

## Nursing Interventions

Preventing Hypovolemia through Control of Bleeding:

- Render emergency care for bleeding.
  - Apply pressure and cold on the area for 10 to 15 minutes to allow clot formation. This ought to be done particularly after venipuncture or injection.
  - Place fibrin foam or absorbable gelatin foam in the wound.
  - Suturing and cauterization ought to be avoided.
  - Immobilize the affected part and elevate above the level of the heart.
  - Administer recombinant factor VIII or factor IX coagulation concentrate.
- Avoid fast administration to minimize the possibility of transfusion reaction; usually 2 to 3 mL/minute; consult package inserts.
- Cryoprecipitate and fresh frozen plasma are not suggested due to their lack of viral inactivation treatment.
- Stop the transfusion if hives, headaches, tingling, chills, flushing, or fever occurs.
  - Apply fibrinolytic agents to wound for oral bleeding.
  - Keep child quiet during treatment to decrease pulse and rate of bleeding.
  - Monitor vital signs and treat for shock if child becomes hypotensive.

Rendering Protection Against Bleeding:

- Avoid rectal temperatures; insert thermometer probe gently and use axillary, oral (if age appropriate), or external ear route.

- Avoid injections if possible.
  - Administer medications orally whenever possible.
  - Subcutaneous route is preferred over I.M.
  - Apply pressure to injection site for 10 to 15 minutes. Then apply a pressure dressing with self-adhesive gauze (Coban).
- Maintain a safe environment and teach parents safety measures.
  - Pad crib or bed rails.
  - Inspect toys for sharp or rough edges.
  - Offer finger foods and fluids in plastic or paper containers.
  - Supervise small children when they are ambulatory.
  - Use protective devices that the child brings from home. (Many children wear helmets and knee and elbow pads.)
  - Continually assess environment for potential hazards.
  - No straws or sharp eating utensils.
  - No hard candy, suckers, or candy canes.

### Drug Alert

Children with haemophilia shouldn't receive aspirin or compounds containing aspirin because this medication affects platelet function and prolongs bleeding time.

Preserving Mobility

- Treat haemarthrosis or muscle bleed as soon as possible.
- Render supportive care for haemarthrosis.
  - Immobilize the joint in a position of slight flexion.
  - Elevate the affected part above the level of the heart.
  - Apply ice packs. Later, after active bleeding has stopped, apply heat to promote absorption of blood.
- For severe haemarthroses, continue immobilization through casting, if essential, and prevent weight bearing on the affected limb.
- For less severe haemarthroses, start gentle, passive exercise 48 hours after the acute phase to prevent joint stiffness and fibrosis. Progress to active exercises.
- Administer short course of corticosteroids as ordered to relieve inflammation.

- Refer for physical therapy if persistent deformity or if crutches, braces, splints, or specialized treatments are required.

## ENDOCRINE DISORDERS

Endocrine dysfunction in children regularly leads to altered development and growth. Accurate nursing evaluation can help detect variations in growth and developmental patterns, identify such factors as diet and medications that may have an impact on development and growth, and obtain information about compliance and understanding of treatment.

### JUVENILE DIABETES MELLITUS

Diabetes mellitus type 1 (Type 1 diabetes, Type I diabetes, T1D, T1DM, IDDM, juvenile diabetes) is a form of diabetes mellitus. Type 1 diabetes is an autoimmune disease that results in destruction of insulin-producing beta cells of the pancreas. Thus far, such destruction has been permanent, but there is informed speculation that reversing the immune system malfunction may allow recuperation of beta cell function.

Lack of insulin causes an increase of fasting blood glucose (around 70-120 mg/dL in the healthy people) that begins to appear in the urine above the renal threshold (about 190-200mg/dl in most people), thus connecting to the symptom by which the disease was identified in antiquity, sweet urine. Glycosuria or glucose in the urine causes the patients to urinate more regularly, and drink more than usual (polydipsia). Classically, these were the characteristic symptoms which prompted discovery of the disease.

Type 1 has been lethal unless treatment with exogenous insulin, usually via injections which replaces the missing hormone formerly produced by the now non-functional beta cells in the pancreas. In recent years, pancreas transplants have also been used to treat Type 1 diabetes. Islet cell transplant is also being investigated and has been attained in mice and rats, but not clinically in humans. Use of stem cells to regenerate beta cells seems to be a future possibility, but has yet to be demonstrated even in laboratories as of 2008.

Type 1 diabetes (formerly known as "childhood", "juvenile" or "insulin-dependent" diabetes) is not exclusively a childhood problem; the adult incidence of Type 1 is noteworthy - many adults who contract Type 1 diabetes are misdiagnosed with Type 2 due confusion on this point.

There is presently no clinically helpful preventive measure against developing Type 1 diabetes, although a vaccine has been proposed and anti-antibody approaches are also being investigated. Most people who develop Type 1 were otherwise healthy and of a healthy weight on onset, but they can lose weight rapidly and dangerously, if not promptly diagnosed. Though the cause of Type 1 diabetes is still not fully understood, and diet and exercise may help, the immune system damage is characteristic of Type 1.

The most definite laboratory test to distinguish Type 1 from Type 2 diabetes is the C-peptide assay, which is a measure of endogenous insulin production since external insulin has not (to date) included -peptide. However, C-peptide is not absent in Type 1 diabetes till insulin production has fully ceased, which may take months. The presence of anti-islet antibodies (to Glutamic Acid Decarboxylase, Insulinoma Associated Peptide-2 or insulin), or lack of insulin resistance, determined by a glucose tolerance test, would also be suggestive of Type 1. Many Type 2 diabetics continue to produce insulin internally, and all have some degree of insulin resistance.

Testing for GAD 65 antibodies has been proposed as an improved test for differentiating between Type 1 and Type 2 diabetes as it appears that the immune system malfunction is connected with their presence.

## Pathophysiology

The cause of Type 1 diabetes is still not fully understood. Some theorize that Type 1 diabetes is in general a virally triggered autoimmune response in which the immune system's attack on virus infected cells is also directed against the beta cells in the pancreas. The autoimmune attack may be triggered by reaction to an infection, for instance by one of the viruses of the Coxsackie virus family or German measles, though the evidence is inconclusive. In Type 1, pancreatic beta cells in the Islets of Langerhans are destroyed or damaged adequately to effectively abolish endogenous insulin production. This etiology distinguishes Type 1's origin from Type 2. It should also be noted that the use of insulin in treating a patient doesn't mean that patient has Type 1 diabetes; the type of diabetes a patient has is determined only by the cause -- fundamentally by whether the patient is insulin resistant (Type 2) or insulin deficient without insulin resistance (Type 1).

This vulnerability is not shared by everyone, for not everyone infected by the suspected organisms develops Type 1 diabetes. This has suggested presence of a genetic vulnerability and there is indeed an observed inherited tendency to develop Type 1. It has been traced to particular HLA genotypes, although the connection between them and the triggering of an auto-immune reaction is still poorly understood. Wide-scale genetic studies have shown links between genetic vulnerabilities for type 1 diabetes and Multiple Sclerosis and Crohn's Disease.

Some researchers believe that the autoimmune response is regulated by antibodies against cow's milk proteins. A large retrospective controlled study published in 2006 strongly suggests that infants who were never breastfed had a risk for developing Type 1 diabetes twice that of infants who were breastfed for at least three months. The mechanism, if any, is not understood. No connection has been established between autoantibodies, antibodies to cow's milk proteins, and Type 1 diabetes. A subtype of Type 1 (identifiable by the presence of antibodies against beta cells) typically develops slowly and so is frequently confused with Type 2. In addition, a small proportion of Type 1 cases have the hereditary condition maturity onset diabetes of the young (MODY) which can also be confused with Type 2.

Vitamin D in doses of 2000 IU per day given during the first year of a child's life has been connected in one study in Northern Finland (where intrinsic production of Vitamin D is low because of low natural light levels) with an 80% reduction in the risk of getting Type 1 diabetes later in life. The causal connection, if any, is obscure.

Some suggest that deficiency of Vitamin D3 (one of several related chemicals with Vitamin D activity) may be a significant pathogenic factor in Type 1 diabetes independent of geographical latitude, and so of available sun intensity.

Some chemicals and drugs preferentially destroy pancreatic cells. Vacor (N-3-pyridylmethyl-N'-p-nitrophenyl urea), a rodenticide introduced in 1976, selectively destroys pancreatic beta cells, ensuing in Type 1 diabetes after accidental or intentional ingestion. Zanosar is the trade name for streptozotocin, an antibiotic and antineoplastic agent used in chemotherapy for pancreatic cancer; it also kills beta cells, ensuing in loss of insulin production. Other pancreatic problems, including trauma, pancreatitis or tumors (either malignant or benign), can also lead to loss of insulin production.

The exact cause(s) of Type 1 diabetes are not yet fully understood, and research on those mentioned, and others, continues.

In December 2006, researchers from Toronto Hospital for Sick Children published research that shows a link between type I diabetes and the immune and nervous system. Using mice, the researchers discovered that a control circuit exists between insulin-producing cells and their associated sensory (pain-related) nerves. It's being proposed that faulty nerves in the pancreas could be a cause of type I diabetes.

## Treatment

Type 1 is treated with insulin replacement therapy - usually by injection or insulin pump, along with attention to dietary management, typically including carbohydrate tracking, and careful monitoring of blood glucose levels using Glucose meters.

Untreated Type 1 diabetes can lead to one form of diabetic coma, diabetic ketoacidosis, which can be disastrous. At present, insulin treatment must be continued for life; this may change when better treatment, or a cure, becomes clinically available. Continuous glucose monitors have been developed which can alert patients to the presence of dangerously high or low blood sugar levels, but the lack of widespread insurance coverage (certainly in the US) has limited the impact these devices have had on clinical practice so far.

In more extreme cases, a pancreas transplant can restore proper glucose regulation. However, the surgery and accompanying immunosuppression needed is believed to be by many doctors to be more dangerous than continued insulin replacement therapy, and is consequently frequently used only as a last resort (like when a kidney must also be transplanted, or in cases where the patient's blood glucose levels are extremely volatile).

Experimental replacement of beta cells (by transplant or from stem cells) is being investigated in several research programs and may become clinically available in the future. Thus far, beta cell replacement has only been performed on patients over age 18, and with tantalizing successes amidst nearly universal failure.

### *Pancreas Transplantation*

Pancreas transplants are in general suggested if a kidney transplant is also essential. The reason for this is that introducing a new kidney calls for taking immunosuppressive drugs anyway, and this allows the introduction of a new, functioning pancreas to a patient with diabetes without any extra immunosuppressive therapy. However, pancreas transplants alone can be wise in patients with extremely labile type 1 diabetes mellitus.

### Islet Cell Transplantation

Islet cell transplantation is expected to be less invasive than a pancreas transplant which is presently the most commonly used approach in humans.

In one variant of this procedure, islet cells are injected into the patient's liver, where they take up residence and start to produce insulin. The liver is expected to be the most reasonable choice because it is more accessible than the pancreas, and islet cells seem to produce insulin well in that environment. The patient's body, however, will treat the new cells just as it would any other introduction of foreign tissue, unless a method is developed to produce them from the patient's own stem cells or there is an identical twin available who can donate stem cells. The immune system will attack the cells as it would a bacterial infection or a skin graft. Thus, patients now also need to undergo treatment involving immunosuppressants, which reduce immune system activity.

Recent studies have shown that islet cell transplants have progressed to the point that 58% of the patients in one study were insulin independent one year after islet cell transplant. Ideally, it would be best to use islet cells which will not provoke this immune reaction, but investigators are also looking into placing them within a protective housing which enables insulin to flow out and nutrients to flow in while protecting the islets from immune system attack via white blood cells.

## ORTHOPEDIC DISORDERS

## FRACTURES

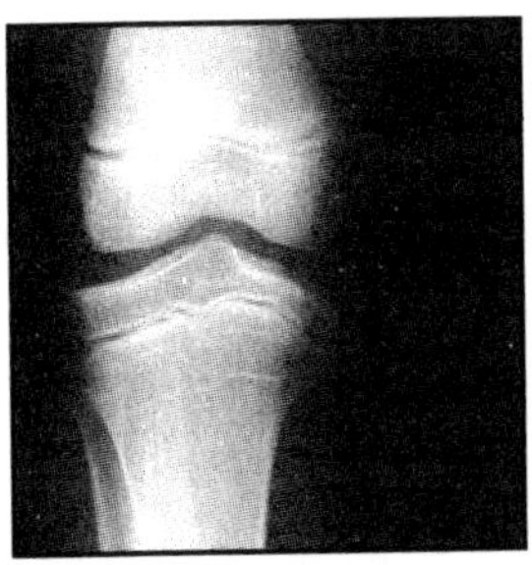

*Fig. Fractures*

A fracture is a break or disruption in the continuity of bone. Fractures in children differ from those in adults because of the differences in anatomy, biomechanics, and physiology of the child's skeleton as compared to that of an adult. The incidence of musculoskeletal injuries sustained by children and adolescents has increased significantly in the past 2 decades. Males have a 40% chance of sustaining a fracture before age 16 while females have a 25% chance.

## Nursing Evaluation

- Follow the basic evaluation for the trauma victim.
- Obtain history from child, parents, and others to include accident or trauma details, noting the position of the extremity at impact.
- Perform physical examination for location of deformity, swelling, ecchymosis, and pain; vital signs; and neurovascular evaluation.
- Assess child's support mechanisms/social situation with consideration of discharge requirements.

## Nursing Diagnoses

- Acute Pain associated with tissue trauma and reflex muscle spasms secondary to fracture
- Ineffective Tissue Perfusion: Peripheral associated with swelling and immobilization
- Impaired Skin Integrity associated with mechanical trauma (e.g., fixation device, traction, casts, other orthopedic devices)
- Ineffective Coping associated with separation from family and home
- Impaired Physical Mobility associated with fracture and external immobilization device (e.g., cast, splint, external fixator)
- Bathing/Hygiene/Feeding/Toileting Self-Care Deficit associated with external devices (e.g., cast, splint)
- Risk for Infection associated with trauma (fracture) and surgery
- Risk for Peripheral Neurovascular Dysfunction associated with restrictive envelope secondary to cast or splint

## Nursing Interventions

- Monitor and assess pain level using an age-appropriate pain scale (eg, Oucher or FACES scale).
- Correctly position, align, and support affected body part.
- Administer analgesics as indicated and monitor effectiveness of analgesia.

- Use nontraditional methods of pain relief-music therapy, diversionary activities, relaxation techniques, therapeutic touch, play therapy.
- Regularly assess perfusion of limb by checking temperature, colour, sensation, and pulses.
- Elevate extremity above heart level to prevent oedema.
- Encourage movement of digits on affected limb.
- Remove compressive bandages (e.g., elastic bandages, splints) that restrict flow of circulation.

## HIP DISLOCATION

Previously referred to as congenital dislocation of the hip, developmental dysplasia of the hip (DDH) is now the accepted term used to describe abnormalities of the developing hip including subluxation, dislocation, and dysplasia of the hip joint. DDH may be linked with other congenital anomalies; its incidence is 1 in 1,000 live births. It is geographically and ethnically variable. Bilateral involvement occurs in more than 50% of cases, and the left hip is more regularly involved than the right hip. Females are afflicted eight times more regularly than males.

### Nursing Evaluation

- Obtain a family history, including hip pathology.
- Obtain an obstetric history for presence of risk factors, like breech presentation and first-born status.
- Perform a physical evaluation for ROM, appearance of Trendelenburg's sign, Barlow test, Ortolani test, and examination for asymmetric thigh folds.
- Assess family's response to the diagnosis.

### Nursing Diagnoses

- Risk for Impaired Parenting associated with ineffective adjustment to stressors linked with a diagnosis of DDH and the prescribed therapeutic regimen
- Risk for Impaired Skin Integrity associated with perineal soiling secondary to confinement in an orthopaedic device (e.g., Pavlik harness, hip-spica cast)
- Impaired Physical Mobility associated with external device (e.g., hip-spica cast)

## Nursing Interventions

- Explain the condition and treatment in terms the family can understand.
- Encourage holding the child with abduction of the hips while handling.
- Advise parents to avoid swaddling the infant.
- Reassure parents that effective outcome depends on early intervention and compliance.
- Demonstrate application of Pavlik harness and make sure that parents know and feel comfortable in applying it.
- Stress importance of keeping follow-up appointments and strict compliance with prescribed treatment.
- Render parents with the name and number of a contact person if they have concerns about their child's care.
- Stimulate the child with games and activities to exercise upper body and feet as able.
- Turn the child regularly and encourage ambulation as able. Support the head and legs to reposition.
- Encourage deep-breathing exercises at time interval to prevent atelectasis and hypostatic pneumonia. Children can blow bubbles, party favors, and cotton balls across the table as appropriate.
- Encourage fluids and a high-fibre diet to prevent constipation.

## CLUBFOOT

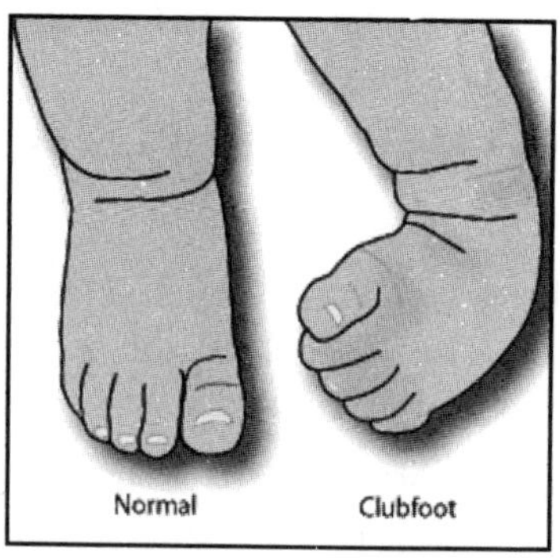


*Fig. Clubfoot*

Clubfoot is a congenital anomaly characterized by a three-part deformity of the foot, consisting of inversion of the heel (hindfoot varus), adduction and supination of the forefoot, and ankle equinus. Other congenital disorders of the foot and ankle occur but are less common. Incidence of clubfoot is 1 to 3 in 1,000 live births. It is bilateral in 50% of afflicted children and occurs in males 2?½ times as regularly as it does in females.

## Nursing Evaluation

- Obtain a family history of foot deformities.
- Obtain an obstetric history for risk factors.
- Perform a physical evaluation for presence of other anomalies and classic foot position and ROM. If late presentation, perform a thorough neurologic examination to rule out causative factors.
- Assess family coping and resources available for lengthy treatment.

## Nursing Diagnoses

- Risk for Impaired Parenting associated with ineffective adjustment to stressors linked with a diagnosis of clubfoot and the therapeutic regimen
- Risk for Impaired Skin Integrity associated with serial casting
- Ineffective Tissue Perfusion: Peripheral associated with postoperative oedema and/or casting
- Acute Pain associated with tissue and muscle trauma secondary to surgery

## Nursing Interventions

- Render an accurate description of deformity and the importance of treatment in terms the parents can understand.
- Render opportunity for parents to verbalize questions and concerns.
- Reinforce causative factors and the fact that it was not anyone's fault that the child has clubfoot.
- Encourage parents to hold and play with child and participate in care.
- Render parents with a contact family that has been through the treatment process for support.
- Assess fit of cast, splint, orthotic device, or special shoes. Advise parents that because of fast growth rate of infant, the

cast or splint may need to be replaced to prevent skin breakdown.

- Assess and teach evaluation of excessive pressure on skin-redness, excoriation, foul odour from underneath cast, or pain.
- Perform frequent neurovascular assessments after surgery, including colour, warmth, sensation, capillary refill, pulses, and presence of pain.
- Elevate the extremity to prevent oedema in the postoperative period.
- Protect and assess foot for injury.
- Assess for signs of discomfort, like irritability, crying, poor feeding and sleeping, tachycardia, and increased blood pressure.
- Administer analgesics on a regular basis for 24 to 48 hours after surgery.
- Render comfort measures like soft music, pacifier, teething ring, rocking and cuddling with parent.
- Encourage parents to administer analgesics after discharge from hospital (when required). Discuss dosage and administration and dispel misconceptions about addiction.

## DISORDERS OF SKIN

### IMPETIGO CONTAGIOSA

Impetigo contagiosa, such as most of the other skin diseases to be described, affects persons of all ages but is seen chiefly in children. It has no common name. While not contagious in the true sense of the word it is highly infectious.

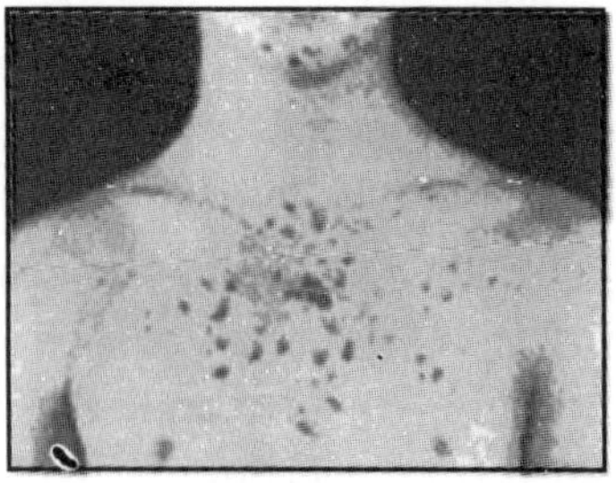

*Fig. Impetigo Contagiosa*

The lesions are crusts (scabs) varying in colour from yellow to dark red. They are sometimes more than an inch in diameter but usually smaller and in most cases are limited to the exposed parts of the body (face, ears, neck, and sometimes the hands), from one or two to a dozen being present ordinarily. There is practically no itching, burning, or other subjective symptom.

The disease is because of bacteria of a variety which are generally present somewhat on the skin of all persons. The bacteria gain access into the skin at the site of an abrasion, like might occur from a scratch or a cut or as a result of picking the face with dirty finger nails. The disorder may occur as a result of a "running" nose or ear. It spreads rapidly, several lesions (sores) being present within a few days or a week after the disease is contracted. Several or all of the children in a family may become likewise affected if they use a common towel or wash cloth, play together, or have other intimate contact.

Cleanliness, especially in the sense of free use of soap and water, and avoidance of picking at the skin are of importance in the prevention of this disease. Each child should use his own towel, wash cloth, comb, and brush. A scratch or cut ought to be treated as soon as possible with mercurochrome or some other non-irritating antiseptic. Though the disorder usually clears up within a week if an ammoniated mercury salve of the proper strength is used, there is no immunity established. The disorder will consequently reappear just as frequently as one becomes infected in the manner described. It is safer to have the child remain at home during the first three of four days of treatment than to instruct him not to associate with other children. The teacher's responsibility is to recognize the disease and at once remove the child who has it from contact with other children.

## PEDICULOSIS

The varieties of lice affect children: (1) the head louse and (2) the body louse.

The head lose, such as the body variety, although easily visible to the naked eye, is seldom seen on the infected person. Rather, one sees its eggs, which are minute, white oval bodies, so-called "nits," deposited on the scalp hairs. They are attached to the hair shafts by a cement substance. A person so afflicted has periodic itching and stinging sensations in the scalp, particularly in the back half. One examination, one commonly sees scratch marks on the back of the neck in addition to nits on some of the scalp hairs.

The disorder is regularly seen in children whose home hygienic conditions are the best, the disorder ensuing from contact with children who are less clean.

Treatment consists in washing the scalp with kerosene, care being taken to protect the surrounding skin with a towel or band of cloth. When the hair is saturated, it ought to be covered with a bandage or towel, which ought to be allowed to remain on all night. After the kerosene is washed out the next morning with a good soap, one may be certain that all the parasites in addition to most of the eggs are destroyed.

The rest of nits may be destroyed by shampooing the scalp with vinegar, which dissolves the cement substance that holds the eggs fast to the hair. A comb with fine teeth may then be used to carry the nits, loosened from the hair shafts to which they were attached, from the hair and scalp. A soup-and-water shampoo will leave the hair and scalp in a healthy state. Crusted sores of several sizes sometimes form on or near the scalp as the result of infected scratch marks. An ammoniated mercury ointment of the proper strength applied nightly is effective.

The body louse is found less commonly on children than is the head louse. It causes itching of the trunk chiefly but somewhat of the buttocks, things, and arms. The itching is worse during the day, that is, when the infected clothing is in contact with the body. For the most part, the organisms remain in the seams if the clothing. They cause itching and stinging sensations only when they are on tithe body feeding.

Their eggs are deposited partly in the clothing and partly on the fine hairs of the body. Frequently, however, neither the organisms nor the eggs can be seen, but, upon disrobing the afflicted person, one sees parallel rows of long and short linear scratch marks on the areas which are easily accessible to the finger nails, like the shoulders, the outsides of the upper arms and of the thighs, and the sides and other areas of the trunk. Interspersed with these scratch marks are minute red points, which represent small haemorrhages within the skin at the sites of recent bites. In this form of pediculosis also, one sometimes sees secondary infections, like boils and impetigo, which are a result of scratching.

A good scrub bath and a complete change of clothing are usually all that is essential by way of treatment, the infected clothing being boiled when possible of placed in an oven in a temperature high enough to destroy the parasites and their eggs. As soon as the teacher discovers the presence of lice on a child's scalp or body, the child ought to be sent home and the parents advised concerning the necessity of treatment.

One child with lice may cause the infestation of all the other children in the room.

## SCABIES

Scabies is another disorder which is an infection with an animal parasite. While of much the same appearance as lice, the organisms are scarcely visible to the naked eye. They burrow around within the top layer of the skin and produce itching as they move. The itching is worse at night after the body has become warm in bed. There is sometimes considerable itching during the day, however, when the body has become warm from exertion or from an overheated room or the wearing of excessive clothing. Usually there are hundreds or thousands of the parasites on the body before the afflicted person is aware of the fact that he has a skin disease. If one member of a family is affected, the whole family is likely to be.

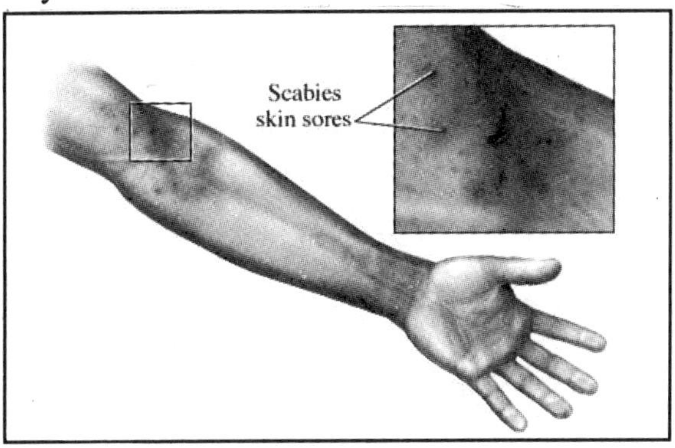


*Fig. Scabies*

The disorder is usually contracted through occupying a bed with an infected person. The parts affected are the trunk and extremities, including the hands, there being no sign of the disorder above the collar line or beneath the ankles except in infants.

The most typical lesions (sores) are seen between the fingers and on the wrists. They appear as small pimples and blisters, on the surface of some of which are seen delicate, black, thread-like, straight or curved lines from an eighth of an inch to a quarter of an inch long. Each line is the path of a parasite in the skin, and it is a furrow filled with dirt, eggs, and excrement of the organism. There are a dozen or more eggs in each furrow, and at one end of it is the parasite. The eggs give rise to new parasites, which crawl out of the surface of the skin. Here the females, which are the only ones that burrow, are fertilized, the males remaining on the surface of the skin. The female perishes after burrowing and laying her eggs. On the regions other than the hands, wrists, genitals, and buttocks, the lesions occur chiefly as scratch marks the size of a pinhead, which can hardly be recognized as lesions of scabies, at least without microscopic examination.

Treatment of scabies consists in applying a sulphur salve for five successive nights. After taking a scrub bath, the affected person should apply the salve from the neck to the ankles, including the hands. A suit of underwear with long sleeves and legs ought to be worn continuously, night and day, it becoming permeated with the sulphur, and thin cotton gloves ought to be worn at night. On the morning following the fifth application of the salve, a cleansing bath is taken and clean clothing put on. Some itching may persist, but it is because of irritation of the skin by the sulphur and ought to be allayed by a few daily applications of olive oil. Scabies may be passed on from one child to another by direct contact. Hence, the teacher must recognize this disease and prevent contact between the infected child and others.

## RINGWORM OF THE SCALP

Ringworm is a disease of the skin, hair, and nails which is produced by numerous varieties of vegetable parasites called "fungi."

In children ringworm is seen chiefly in the scalp, and practically all the cases of ringworm of the scalp are in children. There are, in general speaking, three varieties of ringworm in this area.

The most common type, which constitutes about 95 per cent of the cases, begins at any time during and, in the absence of treatment, disappears spontaneously at the age of puberty. It is highly infectious and is seen spread amongst the playmates of a child who is infected with it. It is consequently advisable that any person afflicted with it be isolated from his fellows. The teacher must recognize the disease and send the infected child home.

This type of ringworm resists treatment by ordinary means, like ointments and other local applications. It begins as one or more patches in which the hairs appear to be nibbled off. In the beginning these areas are about one-fourth of an inch in diameter. They may gradually enlarge and fuse to such an extent as to involve practically the total scalp. As a rule, however, the disorder is limited to from three to a dozen round patches varying in size from a half-inch to an inch and one-half in diameter. Many of the hair stumps in the involved areas have delicate whitish sheaths about them, and the patches have the appearance of having been strewn with ashes, the grayish appearance being because of fine scaling in the areas. There is usually no redness or other sign of inflammation in the patches, and ordinarily there is no itching or other subjective symptom. Permanent baldness in the affected areas doesn't occur in this type of ringworm.

The next most common type of ringworm of the scalp is called "kerion" and, unlike that just described, is moist. Though it is seen most commonly in children, it sometimes occurs in adults. This variety is usually contracted from playing with animals that are infected with the causative organism, most commonly dogs or cats. This variety constitutes only about three per cent of the cases of ringworm of the scalp. Apparently it is not so infectious as the type previously described, but the infected child shouldn't be allowed to attend school till he is pronounced non-infectious by a doctor.

This type usually occurs as from one to three or four swellings varying in size from that of a hazelnut to that of a hen's egg. The swellings are to some extent tender. Not uncommonly the lymph glands of the neck are slightly enlarged. Swellings are soft and feel as although, upon puncture, pus would be evacuated, but they don't contain pus. The hairs in the area are usually broken off at several lengths, and the inflammation present pushes these hairs from their follicles in the course of a few days or weeks. From the gaping follicle mouths a colorless, syrupy fluid exudes. Any hairs in the area can be pulled out such as pins from a pincushion. After a variable period time, usually several weeks, the disorder clears up spontaneously, but proper treatment hastens the disappearance of the lesions and prevents the spread of the infection to other parts of the scalp and to persons with whom the affected person is associated. Scarring, with baldness, usually results from this type of ringworm.

A third type of ringworm of the scalp, the rarest type, occurs as black dots the size of a pinhead or smaller scattered over the scalp. Ordinarily it can be detected only by the expert eye though sometimes it is first noticed by the observant mother or attendant when she is shampooing the child's hair. It causes very little loss of hair and is responsible for no irritation. This type, such as the first described, is of human origin. The black dots mentioned are usually seen even in individuals with light hair. They are produced by the growth of a single hair curled upon itself beneath a small transparent scale. No scarring results. Isolation of the infected child ought to be accomplished in this type of ringworm.

All the types of ringworm of the scalp described may be linked with lesions on the non-hairy skin though this is exceptional.

## RINGWORM OF THE BODY

Ringworm of the body. - Ringworm of the body usually occurs as from one to a dozen red rings varying in size from a half-inch to an inch and one-half in diameter. In the beginning the lesions are usually solid discs, but within a few days after their appearance they clear in the centre, thus forming a circle. This characteristic is responsible for the common name of the disorder. The lesions may be of the dry type, there being only redness and scaling, or they may be of the moist type, in which case there are little blisters at the outer edge of the ring, the blisters later becoming small crusts.

One type occurs with about the same frequency as the other, and in any given instance the lesions are totally of one type. There are itching and other sensations in the body eruption, but they are usually mild. Ringworm of the body is commonly but not always contracted from the handling of cats, dogs, and other pets whose hairs are infected with the fungi. If there are several children in the family, usually more than one is affected and not uncommonly the mother or nurse also. This type of ringworm responds readily to the proper local preparations. Because the infected child may pass the condition on to others, he ought to be isolated till treated.

## RINGWORM OF THE HANDS, FEET, CROTCH, AND ARMPITS

Ringworm of the hands and feet is deserving of separate description because it has certain characteristics not seen in the other types of ringworm of the body. It is most frequently contracted from walking barefoot on floors infected with the causative organism, notably those in shower rooms and gymnasiums. Usually this variety begins between and under the toes as an itching, splitting, and maceration of the skin. Later, blisters usually appear on the soles and sides of the feet. These blisters are deep-seated they tend not to rupture spontaneously but to dry up and leave brownish thickenings at their sites. The disorder is almost invariably worse in hot weather. Itching is usually periodically intense, and, as a result of scratching the feet, the individual transfers of the organisms to the other parts of the body on which they will grow. It is a peculiar fact that the organism will grow readily only on the feet, hands, crotch, and armpits. The eruption seen on the hands is almost identical with that occurring on the feet.

The disorder occurs in the crotch and armpits as diffuse, red, scaling areas which itch intensely and have the appearance of irritation produced by changing. As it occurs in these areas, it is the disorder referred to as "gym itch." Fortunately, ringworm of the hands, feet, crotch, and armpits is usually easily remedied.

Ringworm of the beard and ringworm of the nails need not to be discussed here. Both are extremely rare, and the former is hardly to be expected in young persons. Because it is at times possible for the doctor, to say nothing of the layman, to have some question about the diagnosis of ringworm upon mere observation, it is essential, before treatment is instituted, to demonstrate the causative organisms under the microscope. This is a very simple procedure and can be accomplished in a few minutes by one skilled in this work. If there is any question in the teacher's mind about any skin lesion, it is her responsibility to have the particular child isolated till a diagnosis is made.

## WARTS

There is no basis for the popular belief that warts are contracted from the handling of toads. Of the numerous varieties of warts, there are but a few types that need be mentioned here. Everyone is familiar with the common type of wart that is seen especially on the hands of school children. It must be added, however, that this lesion is not uncommon in adults. It is characterized by from one to a dozen or more well-elevated, horny thickenings the size of a match head or larger which occur on any and all surfaces of the fingers and hands.

Though these lesions are usually responsible for no discomfort, they frequently become inflamed when they are so located that they are regularly injured. When they appear around the under the nails, they are especially rebellious to treatment. Such cases are probably frequently the result of improper manicuring.

This, such as most of the other types of warts, is an infection by an organism so small that it can't be detected by the most powerful microscope. It is perhaps the same organism that is responsible for the painful wart which appears of the soles of the feet, the so-called "plantar" wart. In the latter case the organism usually gains entrance into the skin through such an abrasion as might be produced by a nail in the shoe or from an injury ensuing from going barefooted.

There is good evidence that some gymnasiums are infested with this organism because not uncommonly many children in a single school are seen with this painful type of wart. It can be treated satisfactorily only by a competent doctor, X-ray treatments frequently being essential, a procedure to be entrusted only to one skilled in this work.

Warts on the hand are usually most satisfactorily cared for by freezing them with carbon-dioxide snow after they have been well softened. One shouldn't pick at warts. Picking them will not cure them, and it will spread them. The old practice of applying nitric acid and other strong caustics to these growths ought to be discouraged. Such treatment frequently leaves disfiguring scars, and the infection so severe as to cause blood poisoning may result.

Another type of wart not infrequently seen in school children appears on the back of the hands, and more rarely on the cheeks and forehead, as numerous flat, smooth, shiny, flesh-colored to light brown thickenings which vary in size from that of a pinhead to that of a match head. These thickenings are devoid of all subjective symptoms. Though this type of wart is infectious, there is little danger of its being transmitted from one person to another. It sometimes occurs along with the common type of wart and, like it, tends to resist treatment.

The teacher's responsibility towards the child in such cases is to insist on proper treatment in order to prevent spread of the condition. If many children are suffering from warts on the feet, the floors, particularly the floor of the gymnasium, ought to be scrubbed well with soap and water and disinfectants employed.

## ACNE VULGARIS

Acne vulgaris, commonly referred to as pimples and blackheads, is usually most marked during the teens, the period at which all the glands of the body are developing and are overactive. Probably as many as 90 per cent of all young persons have acne to some degree. The disorder is manifested by large or small pimples and blackheads, seen chiefly on the face, forehead, neck, back, chest, and outer surfaces of the arms, and commonly it is linked with and excessive oiliness of the skin and with considerable dandruff of the scalp.

It is supposedly caused primarily by an infection of the fat glands of the skin, and, although not of internal origin, it is regulated by internal factors. Anything that decreases the person's normal vitality tends to aggravate the acne, whether this is constipation, faulty diet, anaemia, inadequate sleep, or improper hygiene.

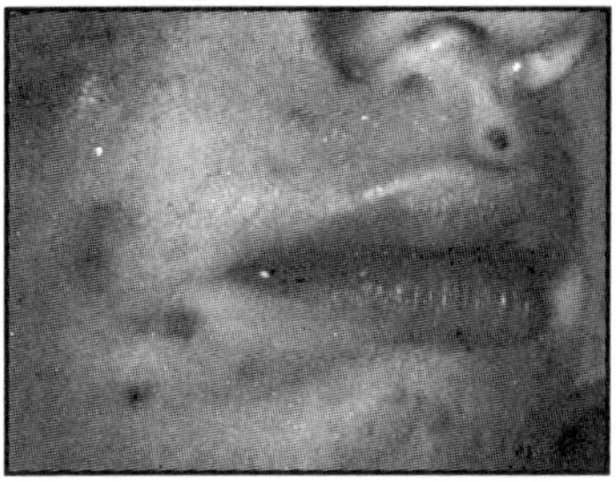

*Fig. Acne Vulgaris*

In young women it is regularly aggravated by the menstrual period. In such cases the eruption not uncommonly practically clears up shortly after the menstrual period only to become aggravated shortly before the time of the next period. The disorder is seen commonly even in individuals who are meticulous in their hygiene. All cases of acne ought to be correctly treated to avoid subsequent scarring and to afford the afflicted person a minimum of embarrassment. Treatment ought to be given despite the fact that there is a tendency toward eventual spontaneous cure of the disorder. It seldom persists long after the person has reached the age of twenty years.

All persons with acne should avoid an excess of sweets, fried foods, highly seasoned articles of diet, and indigestible foods. They should eat three meals a day at regular hours and avoid coffee, alcoholics, and other stimulating drinks. They ought to be instructed not to take hot baths but to take tepid baths as desired for hygienic purposes and a cold shower or a cold tub every morning. Fresh aid, sunshine, enough rest and sleep, and exercise in moderation are significant. The bowels ought to be influenced by diet alone. Personal cases vary so greatly in their characteristics that any medicinal treatment ought to be carried out only under the direction of a doctor.

The teacher must distinguish between acne and skin diseases that are infectious. An attempt must be made to prevent the afflicted person from becoming self-conscious due to the condition because it appears at that time of life when the average person wants to look his best.

## BOILS AND CARBUNCLES

Boils, scientifically known as "furuncles," the condition as "furunculosis," occur in persons of all ages and are infections of the hair follicles and their attached fat glands. The organisms responsible for boils are generally present on the skin of all persons, but for some reason they find the skin of one person a better place to grow in than that of another. Amongst the predisposing factors are diabetes, changing of the skin and other forms of external irritation, in addition to the factors enumerated under acne.

Boils occur as large, hard, painful, tender pimples, and upon palpation it can be ascertained that the involved area is much larger than it appears to be, the tissue around the boil in a field an inch or more in diameter usually being hard. In a person with furunculosis there are usually only two or three lesions present at a time. Because the person spreads the infection on himself, there is not uncommonly a history of the presence of fifteen or twenty boils before a doctor is consulted. About a week after a boil makes its appearance, it becomes soft and exudes pus, and in the course of the next week a "core" comes from it. From this time on healing is fast.

Boils differ from carbuncles only in that in the case of the former a single hair follicle is involved and the lesion consequently has but a single opening, whereas in the case of the latter a number of hair follicles are involved and the lesion consequently has several openings. It is apparent, consequently, that the carbuncle is the more formidable lesion and consequently is responsible for much more pain and tenderness and calls for a longer period of time to heal. The most dangerous boils and carbuncles are those situated about the nose and upper lip.

Till further essential instructions and treatment are received from a doctor, it is well for a person with boils to apply to the lesions a hot wet dressing of boric acid or epsom salts, a teaspoonful of either to a pint of hot water, the dressings to be applied for ten or fifteen minutes two or three times a day. The normal measures outlined under the discussion of acne are of importance in the treatment of boils and carbuncles. Vaccines, internal medication, ointments, and other measures may also be indicated. Needless to say, if the patient has diabetes, this disease should receive proper attention.

## EYE PROBLEMS

Infectious processes of the eye include conjunctivitis, orbital or periorbital cellulitis, and hordeolum. They are characterized by inflammation and tissue damage caused by microbes, like bacteria, viruses, or Chlamydia trachomatis. Conjunctivitis is a common problem, affecting almost all children at some time or another.

## Nursing Alert

A child who has a painful red eye ought to be referred promptly for medical assessment because this may indicate herpetic infection or damage to the cornea.

## Nursing Evaluation

- Assess nature and extent of symptoms and their effect on child's activities.
- Assess visual acuity.
- Determine resources available to family for treatment.

## Nursing Diagnoses

- Risk for Infection (transmission) associated with hand-to-hand or hand-to-object contact
- Acute Pain associated with tissue swelling, inflammation, and light sensitivity

## Nursing Interventions

- Perform or teach proper cleansing of drainage.
  - — Use warm water or saline and a disposable applicator, like cotton balls or gauze.
  - — Use a separate applicator for each eye.
  - — Wipe from inner to outer canthus to avoid contamination.
- Teach self-care measures to prevent spread to others.
  - — Observe good hand-washing practices.
  - — Wipe eyes and nose with tissues and dispose promptly.
  - — Avoid rubbing eyes to prevent spread to other eye.
- Administer and teach proper instillation of eyedrops or ointment.
- Administer oral or I.V. antibiotics as indicated.
- Apply warm compresses to affected area.
- Suggest darkened room and sunglasses for patients with photophobia.
- Administer an analgesic as indicated.
- Advise of ways to prevent transmission to others.
  - — Don't share washcloths or towels.
  - — Avoid swimming till infection is resolved.
  - — The child can return to school after having received antibiotic treatment for 24 hours.

  - Dispose of contaminated items in proper receptacles.
- Advise parents of indications for reevaluation by healthcare provider.
  - Lack of response to antibiotic treatment.
  - Increase in swelling and tenderness.
  - Eye pain.
  - Worsening of visual acuity.
  - Development of extra symptoms like fever.

## CONGENITAL PROBLEMS OF THE EYES

Congenital problems of the eye include structural defects present at birth or developing soon thereafter. These are usually genetically transmitted. They include cataract, dacryostenosis, glaucoma, ptosis, and strabismus.

### Nursing Evaluation

- Assess for red light reflex, particularly in neonates. Absence or asymmetry of the red light reflex may indicate congenital cataract or an intraocular tumour.
- Inspect the eyes for redness of conjunctiva, cloudiness of the cornea, excessive tearing, eyelids that partially occlude the pupil, or obvious misalignment, which render clues to congenital eye problems.
- Assess visual acuity routinely in infants and children. Changes in acuity may be the first manifestation of a problem or indication of effectiveness of treatment.
- Perform Hirschberg's test for symmetry of the pupillary light reflexes to help detect strabismus. Generally, the light reflexes are in the same position in each pupil when a light is shone on the bridge of the nose, but asymmetrical reflection will occur with strabismus (positive Hirschberg's test).
- Perform the cross cover test to detect latent strabismus caused by weak eye muscles. When the patient is fixated on an object approximately 12 inches (30.5 cm) away and one eye is covered, observe the uncovered eye. If movement occurs, this eye most likely has strabismus. When the eye with strabismus is covered, it drifts out of position and can be seen snapping back rapidly when uncovered.

## Nursing Diagnoses

- Disturbed Sensory Perception (Visual), associated with reduction in visual acuity
- Disturbed Body Image associated with the need for patch or glasses
- Risk for Injury associated with reduced visual acuity and modified depth perception
- Delayed Development and growth associated with altered visual stimulation and possible overprotective behaviour of parents

## Nursing Interventions

- Participate in visual acuity problem identification and encourage prompt treatment to minimize functional impairment.
  - — Neonates ought to be examined in the nursery to detect congenital eye problems.
  - — All children ought to be screened for visual acuity and strabismus. In young children, this is accomplished by physical examination and evaluation of developmental milestones (ie, looks at mother's face, smiles responsively, reaches for objects). By ages 3 to 5, most children can cooperate for performance of accurate visual acuity screening tests.
- Encourage and assist parents in obtaining corrective lenses for child.
- Encourage and assist parents in rendering usual experiences for child to attain maximum potential:
  - — Assist parents in locating and accessing resources, like financial assistance, special education in Braille, or parent support groups.
  - — Advise parents of their child's right to a public education.
- Encourage parents to focus on normalization instead of on overprotection. This means having expectations based on the child's abilities instead of disabilities, rendering opportunities for interaction with peers, and making the child's life as usual as possible.
- Encourage acceptance of appearance and emphasize the positive aspects of treatment.

- Encourage the family to be aware of safety in the home, school, and society.
  - Suggest the use of impact-resistant eyeglasses and devices to keep eyeglasses from falling off.
  - Advise the family to maintain a consistent and uncluttered furniture arrangement; notify child of planned changes.
  - Instruct child in the use of a cane or other assistive device.
  - Teach traffic safety and personal security measures.
- Orient visually impaired children in the hospital to the placement of furniture and other objects in their room.
  - Orient child to food placement on meal trays.
  - Assist child with ambulation and use side rails on bed or crib to prevent falls.

## EYE TRAUMA

Eye trauma causes structural damage to the eye and is produced by mechanical force or contact with a corrosive chemical. Some common types of eye trauma are corneal abrasions, blunt trauma, perforating injuries, and chemical injuries. Eye injuries are common amongst children and are usually associated with their involvement in vigorous play activities.

### Nursing Alert

Never remove a penetrating object from the eye. It ought to be stabilized and the eye ought to be shielded with no pressure applied. The other eye ought to be patched and the patient transported by stretcher. The head ought to be elevated 30 degrees to avoid increased IOP, and the child ought to be kept on nothing-by-mouth orders in preparation for surgery.

- Gentle flushing of the affected eyes with water will help remove the offending chemical. This ought to be done from the inner aspect of eye to the outer to prevent contaminated water from flowing into the other eye.
- Antibiotics may be prescribed to prevent infection.
- Further management depends on the nature and extent of the injury.

### Nursing Evaluation

- Obtain history of injury, including the child's account of how the injury occurred, and a description of symptoms experienced.

- Inspect for location and extent of swelling and bruising, asymmetry, or abnormality in appearance of any part of the eye.
- Assess visual acuity and compare with baseline. This should include near and far acuity in each eye. If the patient can't see well enough to read a Snellen chart, assess ability to count fingers or perceive light.

### Nursing Diagnoses

- Acute Pain associated with inflammation, photophobia, or trauma to eye tissue
- Risk for Injury associated with impaired vision and adverse effects of pain medications
- Feeding, Dressing, and Grooming Self-Care Deficit associated with impaired vision and adverse effects of pain medications

### Nursing Interventions

- Apply cold compresses to the affected area to help reduce swelling and discomfort.
- Keep the child's room as dark as possible to help reduce pain for photophobic patients.
- Administer or teach parents to administer analgesics as prescribed.
- Enforce safety measures.
  - — Use of bed side rails.
  - — Assistance with ambulation.
  - — Close observation.

## FUNCTIONAL PROBLEMS

Functional problems of the eye involve impairment of the vision due to refractive errors or disuse of visual pathways. Such problems regularly result in amblyopia-impaired vision in one or both eyes because of poor visual stimulation instead of an organic problem. Abnormal vision screening with referral occurs in 1.2% of 5-year-old patients and increases to 9.1% by the time the child reaches age 13. Amblyopia affects 1% to 3% of the population.

### Nursing Evaluation

- Start visual acuity screening early, in the pre-school years, and whenever a child displays behaviours suggestive of acuity problems.

- Assess Hirschberg's test for symmetry of the pupillary light reflexes routinely, beginning at birth.
- Perform the cross cover test as part of routine eye evaluation as soon as the child can cooperate (as young as age 3).
- Assess the effect of the functional deficit on the child's overall function, including academic progress, self-esteem, and safety.

## Nursing Diagnoses

- Disturbed Sensory Perception (Visual) associated with reduced acuity or inability to use one eye
- Risk for Injury associated with impaired visual acuity or lack of depth perception
- Chronic Low Self-Esteem associated with lowered performance caused by poor vision

## Nursing Interventions

- Encourage the consistent use of corrective lenses as prescribed.
- Teach the parents ways to help develop the child's skills in interpreting information through the senses of hearing, smell, and touch.
  - Familiarize the child with common sounds and smells in the environment. Besides, orient the child to traffic sounds and sounds linked with danger, like animals and speeding vehicles, and instruct the child how to respond.
  - Use voice or touch, instead of facial expressions or gestures, to express emotion.
  - Speak to the child before touching to reduce startling.
  - Allow the child to touch and handle unfamiliar objects to learn about them.
  - Have the child practice such things as retelling stories and giving the home telephone number and address.
  - Explain unfamiliar sounds and smells to the hospitalized child.
- Recommend the use of shatterproof eyeglasses with flexible frames.
- Recommend the use of eye protection on a routine basis because eye trauma can occur unexpectedly. This is particularly significant for children who rely on only one eye.

- Suggest additional protection, like shatterproof goggles or shields, when participating in contact or ball sports and activities.
- Maintain a stable arrangement of furniture in the home, sufficient lighting, and an uncluttered environment to minimize falls.
- Orient hospitalized children to the hospital room and offer assistance when walking.

# EAR PROBLEMS

## EUSTACHIAN TUBE DYSFUNCTION

Eustachian tube dysfunction (ETD) comprises disorders that arise from closure of the eustachian tube, which ventilates the middle ear to equalize pressure on both sides of the tympanic membrane. ETD leads to middle ear effusion. ETD may present as otitis media with effusion (OME), also known as serous otitis; acute otitis media (AOM); and recurrent otitis media. Approximately 91% of children experience one or more episodes of middle ear effusion by the time they are age 2 years.

### Nursing Evaluation

- Assess for etiologic factors that contribute to eustachian tube dysfunction.
- Assess for symptoms of serous otitis and AOM to identify and to document the nature and severity of the illness.
- Assess hearing after the middle ear effusion is resolved. Promptly identify any hearing loss that may have social and educational consequences.
- Assess speech and language development in children who experience recurrent or prolonged infections to determine deficits.
- Assess for effects of illness on family, like sleep deprivation of parents caused by staying up with child at night or decreased attendance at work caused by keeping child out of school.

### Nursing Alert

Prompt identification of speech and language delays is significant in young children because speech and language development is quite fast at this time. The young children may demonstrate fast regression or failure of progression.

## Nursing Diagnoses

- Acute Pain associated with increased pressure in the middle ear
- Disturbed Sensory Perception (Auditory), associated with reduced sound wave conduction
- Impaired Verbal Communication caused by conductive hearing loss

## Nursing Interventions

- Administer and teach parents to administer antibiotics. Render instruction in.
  - — Measurement of correct dosage.
  - — Time of doses.
  - — Importance of administering all doses.
  - — Proper storage and disposal of unused medication.
  - — Adverse effects.
- Administer acetaminophen as directed for pain or fever.
- Apply warm compresses to the external ear.
- Administer analgesic otic drops, if prescribed; usually indicated when no perforation of the tympanic membrane exists.
- Advise elevation of head to facilitate drainage of fluid from the middle ear into the pharynx.
- Teach older children to stimulate opening of their eustachian tubes by yawning or performing Valsalva's maneuver.
- Teach parents to recognize early signs of otitis and to seek prompt treatment.
- Render preoperative and postoperative teaching if ventilation tubes are indicated.
- Stress the importance of the follow-up visit to make sure that otitis has resolved.

## EXTERNAL OTITIS

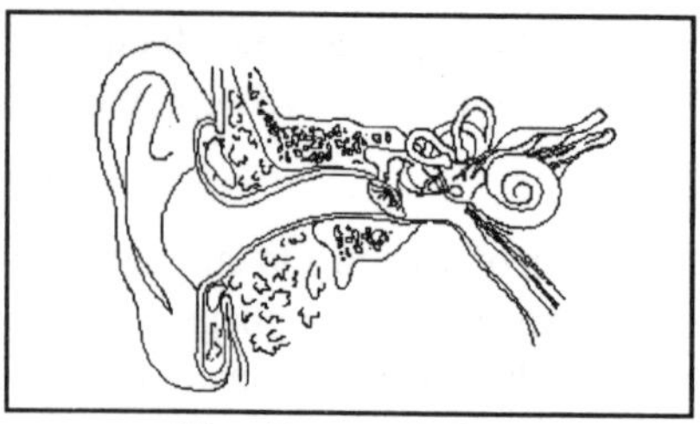

*Fig. External Otitis*

External otitis is inflammation in the external ear canal. It is regularly unilateral but may be bilateral.

### Nursing Evaluation

- Assess severity of symptoms and need for pain relief.
- Assess ear hygiene and the need for earplugs.

### Nursing Diagnosis

- Acute Pain associated with inflammation and irritation of drainage

### Nursing Interventions

- Administer eardrops, or teach parents administration, as prescribed.
  - Have child lie on side with affected ear upward.
  - Instill drops, using caution not to contaminate dropper.
  - Have child maintain position for 5 minutes to facilitate penetration of medication into ear canal.
  - Repeat on other side, if ordered.
- Administer analgesics, like acetaminophen (Tylenol), as directed.
- Suggest application of warm or cold compresses to outer ear to relieve discomfort.
- Regularly clean drainage from area surrounding opening of ear canal to relieve irritation.

## FUNCTIONAL HEARING DISORDERS

Functional hearing disorders arise from problems in the function of the ear. In a quiet environment, the healthy child can hear tones between 0 and 25 decibels. Categories of hearing impairment include slight, 15 to 25 decibels; mild, 25 to 40 decibels; moderate, 40 to 65 decibels; severe, 65 to 95 decibels; and profound, 95 or more decibels. Approximately 5,000 infants are born with moderate to profound bilateral sensorineural hearing loss each year. Factors that place an infant at high risk for hearing loss include low birth weight, family history of hereditary childhood hearing loss, and certain infections, like rubella or bacterial meningitis.

### Nursing Evaluation

- Periodically assess hearing in the child with an identified hearing impairment, to follow up promptly on changes in ability to hear.

- Assess speech and language development regularly so that children may obtain special assistance, as indicated.
- Assess social development and academic progress periodically so that counselling and intervention can be instituted.

## Nursing Diagnoses

- Disturbed Sensory Perception (Auditory), associated with limited ability to hear
- Impaired Verbal Communication associated with inability to hear and imitate speech sounds
- Risk for Injury associated with inability to hear warning sounds of impending danger
- Chronic Low Self-Esteem associated with social and academic difficulties

## Nursing Interventions

- Face the child, use appropriate facial expressions, and make sure the child can see the face distinctly when communicating.
- Approach the child so that the parents can be seen; touch the deaf child on the shoulder to get attention.
- Assist the child in using hearing aid as prescribed.
- Determine usual method of communication: ability to write, using verbal cues, or reading lips. Don't depend on gestures to communicate with child or with a third party who doesn't know sign language.
- Obtain an interpreter, when essential, for children who communicate using sign language. Sufficient communication is particularly significant when rendering health education or when treating children who may have been abused.
- Help the parents of a young child to stimulate and communicate with him or her.
  - — Teach them to use gestures, mime, and nonverbal communication.
  - — Teach them to help the infant to develop watching behaviour by rewarding him with pleasure and praise.
  - — Teach them to talk to the child while looking directly into his eyes and using appropriate facial expressions.

- Advise parents that home safety devices, like smoke detectors, may require visual or tactile alarms (flashing lights or vibration) instead of auditory alarms.
- Encourage the use of other senses to compensate for inability to hear. For instance, the child ought to be particularly careful to look in all directions when crossing the street.
- Don't leave the child alone in an unfamiliar environment without means of communication.
- Render close surveillance and frequent visual contact for the hospitalized child.

## COMMON COMMUNICABLE DISEASES OF CHILDREN

Communicable diseases are illnesses that spread from one person to another. They are also called contagious or infectious diseases. Communicable diseases are caused by germs and tiny bugs. The germs are so small that they can only be seen with a microscope, not with the naked eye. The germs and bugs are categorized as:

- Viruses (e.g., "colds," chicken pox, hepatitis A & B, HIV),
- Bacteria (e.g., "strep," tuberculosis),
- Fungi (e.g., ringworm, thrush), and
- Parasites (e.g., giardia, pinworms, scabies, head lice).

Illnesses caused by bacteria, fungi and parasites always need medical assessment and antibiotic treatment. Many illnesses caused by viruses are mild and go away on their own, but some need medical assessment and treatment.

## SPREAD OF COMMUNICABLE DISEASES

Germs that cause communicable diseases are found in and on people, animals, food, water, air, and dirt. Most of the germs are carried in human "body fluids" - blood, mucus, saliva, vomit, stool, urine, and discharges from the eyes and skin lesions. Most communicable bugs are carried on the skin and hair.

Germs spread when the body fluids of one person get into the body of another person. Most communicable bugs spread by getting onto the skin or hair.

Communicable diseases can be categorized by the way they spread:

- Respiratory diseases (e.g., colds) affect the head and chest. They are spread by:
  - Coughing, sneezing, and breathing,
  - Touching nasal mucus, saliva, and eye discharge.
- Gastrointestinal diseases (e.g., infectious diarrhea) affect the stomach and intestines. They are spread by:
  - Touching stool, vomit, or contaminated surfaces,
  - Eating food contaminated by stool,
  - Drinking or bathing in water contaminated by stool.
- Dermatologic diseases (e.g., ringworm) affect the skin and hair. They are spread by:
  - Touching skin or hair,
  - Sharing items like clothes, hats, towels, and hairbrushes that touch skin or hair.
- Blood-borne diseases (e.g., hepatitis B) affect the total body. They are spread by:
  - Getting blood onto broken skin,
  - Receiving blood transfusions,
  - Sharing needles used for injections, piercing, or tattoos,
  - Having sexual contact that shares body fluids.

The majority of illnesses spread in early childhood programs are respiratory, gastrointestinal, and dermatologic diseases. The spread of blood-borne diseases is extremely rare.

## COMMON AMONGST YOUNG CHILDREN

Young children have frequent illnesses caused by communicable diseases. Studies show that pre-school-age children have symptoms of illness onethird to one-half of the days out of the year.

Young children are more vulnerable to illnesses because their immune systems - the body's natural defenses against disease - are not yet built up. Infants and toddlers tend to get sick more frequently than older children. And when children enter a new childcare setting, they tend to get sick more in the first year. Over time, as children develop and learn, their immune defenses also develop and learn to protect them against diseases and keep them healthier.

For instance, children get frequent colds, but the average number they suffer per year decreases as they get older:

- Infants and toddlers have 6-10 colds/year.
- Pre-school-age children have 3-5 colds/year.
- Older children have 1-3 colds/year.

Communicable diseases spread in early childhood programs because:

- There is close contact amongst many children and germs.
- Young children explore their environment by touching people and things and by putting their hands and objects - and germs - into their mouths.
- Most young children have not yet developed good hygiene practices. They touch their noses, mouths, bottoms, animals, dirt, food, and toys, and frequently forget to wash their hands.
- Surfaces and objects can carry germs. These include toys, tabletops, floors, diapering and toileting areas, sinks, doorknobs, water fountains, sandboxes, and water play tables.
- Teachers and parents also spread germs. Studies of early childhood programs show that the surface most likely to carry germs is the caregiver's hands. In meeting the requirements of many children - wiping runny noses, changing diapers, assisting with toileting, and handling food - proper hygiene practices are sometimes neglected.

## IMPACT

Most of the communicable diseases that children experience, like colds and stomach upsets, are mild. Children are usually sick for a few days and then get better on their own.

Some illnesses, however, are more serious and require medical assessment and treatment. For instance, strep throat needs treatment with antibiotics. Some frequent illnesses can lead to complications. For instance, colds can lead to frequent ear infections in some infants and toddlers, which can lead to hearing loss. Some children with immune problems, like HIV/AIDS, are more susceptible to illnesses. Rarely, communicable diseases like meningitis, measles, and tuberculosis can be disastrous.

The illnesses do not simply spread amongst the children - they also spread to staff, parents, and other family members. Communicable diseases can lead to significant pain and suffering, time missed from school and work, and medical costs for families and staff.

Each person has a distinctive set of beliefs about health and illness. These beliefs are shaped by many factors including cultural background, education, and individual experience. People in the Head Start community - staff, children, parents, and other professionals - have diverse beliefs about communicable diseases, including:

- Beliefs about the causes of illness, for instance, germs, poor hygiene, lowered resistance, weak constitution, emotions and stress, eating bad food, exposure to cold air, evil eye, punishment for sins, hot/cold imbalance, lack of harmony with nature, and fate.
- Practices to maintain health and treat illness, for instance, washing hands, eating certain foods, exercise/rest, bathing/not bathing, taking medicine, drinking teas, injections, prayer, laying on hands, religious ceremonies, hot/cold remedies, acupuncture, cupping, coin rubbing, massage, offerings, and family support.
- Sources of health information and treatment, for instance, physicians, nurses, psychologists, chiropractors, homeopaths, family members, elders, healers, religious leaders, pharmacists, acupuncturists, medicine men, santeros, and curanderos.

## Prevention

Because diseases can be transmitted through many different channels, the best way to prevent their spread is with a comprehensive approach. In addition, because the way to prevent the spread of illness is the same for any infection, providers need to understand and use universal precautions against disease.

These same precautions apply whether the provider is caring for one child or a group of children and whether care is in the child's home, the provider's home, or a child care setting. By consistently following these universal precautions, providers also will avoid the unpleasant situation of focusing on one particular child.

The single most important way to prevent infection is hand washing, a fact that supervisors of care providers cannot stress enough. It is recommended that child care workers wash their hands with a liquid disinfectant soap for several minutes at the beginning of their shift, and for at least thirty seconds between each child that they handle. Other universal rules of hygiene:

- Keep each child's personal grooming articles, clothing, and bed linens separate.

- Clean and sanitize toys, utensils, and equipment frequently.
- Dispose of soiled diapers, tissues, and dressings in covered containers.
- Place changing tables and basins away from the food preparation area, and disinfect them after each use.
- Use a diaper service or disposable diapers, whenever possible.
- Use disposable gloves whenever possible for diapering and handling bodily fluids.
- Make certain open sores on both children and providers are always covered.
- Require a physician's approval before a child with skin eruptions can attend group care.

## Healthy Care Providers

Many care providers get sick frequently, particularly when first starting work, because they are exposed to a wider variety of infectious diseases. Also, caring for others can be stressful. Because stress lowers resistance to illness and contributes to burn-out, which in itself can contribute to illness, administrators should encourage providers to take adequate care of themselves. Providing quality care should be of paramount concern to all administrators, and a healthy care provider is the key to a healthy, happy child care experience for both the children and their families.

Program supervisors can encourage providers to stay healthier by emphasizing the importance of:

- hand washing
- good nutrition
- regular exercise
- sufficient daily rest

Providers also should

- Stay current in their immunizations
- Take scheduled breaks and vacations
- Participate in extracurricular hobbies and activities that do not involve caregiving

Providers who are ill should be taking care of themselves, not someone else. In addition to spreading germs to others, a person who is ill cannot provide the usual quality of care and will take longer to get well without the opportunity to recuperate properly.

# CHILD HEALTH EMERGENCIES

## POISONING

Poisoning is a Paediatric emergency and a thorough knowledge about the nature and magnitude of problem particularly when linked with regional peculiarities is essential. Accidents in the home are much too common, particularly because many can be avoided by taking a few simple precautions. Some of the more serious accidents are poisoning incidents involving children. When young children explore the world, they use all their senses including taste. They typically put everything in their mouth to find out what it is. For this reason, adults must make sure that children don't have access to anything poisonous.

It is surprising just how many ordinary household articles are dangerous in this respect. To make the home safe from poisoning, examine it carefully one room at a time. Identify any potentially unsafe substances and either lock them away or store them somewhere out of the children's reach.

Cleaning materials are usually kept in the kitchen, frequently in a low cupboard under the sink where they are easily accessible to curious children. Potentially dangerous products include:

- All kinds of detergents and cleaning products, which frequently contain chemicals that are poisonous to children.
- Plant fertilizer. This is extremely dangerous.
- Detergents used in automatic dishwashers. These are highly caustic and, consequently, very dangerous if consumed.
- Move these products to a locked cabinet where children can't see or reach them. It's not sufficient to simply store them on a worktop because children are excellent climbers. Buy products with childproof lids wherever possible - but lock them away nonetheless.

Never pour chemicals or detergents into empty soft drink or water bottles. Children may think the bottles still contain the original liquid.

Medicines, cosmetics, creams and lotions contain unsafe substances (like alcohol) that may poison a child.

Many tablets, medicines, herbal remedies and even vitamins are dangerous for children. Remember that children are less tolerant than adults and even a small amount may be poisonous.

Always keep such items in a locked cabinet that the children don't have access to. Put any medicines back in the cabinet promptly after use.

What is poisonous in the living room?

Alcohol is very dangerous for children. Always lock cabinets containing wine and spirits - screwing down the lids tightly is not sufficient. Children are very good at opening things and even a small quantity of alcohol can be unsafe to ayoung child.

Remote controls for electronic equipment may contain small mercury batteries, which can cause poisoning if swallowed.

Cigarettes and tobacco are frequently left lying around. Tobacco, in all forms, is an extremely dangerous poison and just one cigarette stub may poison a child. All kinds of tobacco ought to be kept out of the reach of children.

Many houseplants and garden plants are poisonous if eaten.

A pharmacist can render advice about poisonous plants. If the parents have small children, don't keep any poisonous houseplants - even if the parents place them out of reach, leaves may fall to the floor.

Plant poison frequently causes blisters and/or ulcers in the child's mouth or their tongue may begun swelling.

## TREATMENT

Inactivated charcoal is frequently used in hospital emergency departments as an antidote in cases of poisoning. Large doses are used to prevent the poison being absorbed from the stomach. Inactivated charcoal tablets are available to buy from pharmacies, but these are for the treatment of indigestion and flatulence only and shouldn't be used at home to treat poisoning, as the dose they contain is far too small.

For this reason the parents shouldn't keep charcoal tablets as poisoning treatment in the first-aid kit. The parents should always consult a physician or hospital emergency department in cases of poisoning. In some cases of poisoning the physician will suggest that the parents give the child milk. But only do this if the physician has advised it. Induced vomiting - or forcing the child to throw up - is essential only in some cases of poisoning. Do it only if the parents know exactly what has poisoned the child and the physician has told the parents to go ahead. If the child has swallowed a caustic substance it could be extremely dangerous for them to vomit, so always get medical advice first.

## FOREIGN BODY INGESTION

Foreign body ingestion is the swallowing of an object other than food. This commonly happens in children aged six months to six years who tend to put things into their mouths. Once an object is swallowed, it may get stuck in the esophagus or get trapped in the stomach. The esophagus is the tube that connects the mouth to the stomach. Swallowed objects usually pass through the total digestive tract and out of the anus (rear end) without problems.

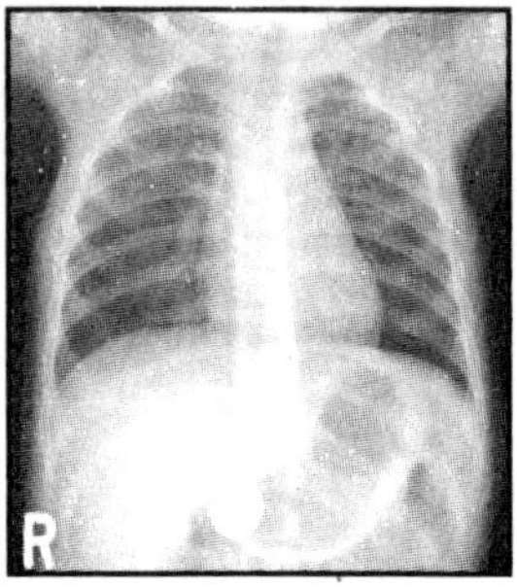


*Fig. Foreign Body Ingestion*

Foreign body ingestion may happen by accident or be done on purpose. Very young children may put anything in their mouth, and swallow the object. Objects may be blunt, sharp, pointed, or poisonous. These may include safety pins, small batteries, needles, school supplies, tacks, seeds, toothpicks, or pieces of toys, glass, or wood. The child may swallow a fish bone or an animal bone while eating. Coins are the most commonly swallowed objects in children.

### Signs and Symptoms

The child may have pain in the neck, throat, chest, or abdomen (belly). He may refuse to eat and have trouble swallowing, gagging, or vomiting (throwing up). He may drool or there may be blood in his saliva. The child may also have breathing problems, like coughing or wheezing (high-pitched sound when breathing).

### Diagnosis

- Barium Swallow: A barium swallow is an x-ray of the child's throat and esophagus. This test may also be called a barium esophagram. The child will be given thick liquid called barium. Barium helps the child's esophagus and stomach show up better on x-rays. Follow the instructions of the child's caregiver before and after the test.

- Computerized Tomography Scan: This test is also called a CT scan. A special x-ray machine uses a computer to take pictures of the child's digestive tract. The child may be given dye by mouth or in an IV before the pictures are taken. The dye may help the child's caregiver see the pictures better. People who are allergic to iodine or shellfish (lobster, crab, or shrimp) may be allergic to some dyes. Tell the caregiver if the child is allergic to shellfish, or has other allergies or medical conditions.
- Endoscopy: Endoscopy is a test that uses a scope to see the inside of the child's digestive tract. A scope is usually made of a long, bendable tube with a light on the end of it. A camera may be hooked to the scope to take pictures. During an endoscopy, caregivers will look for the foreign body. Caregivers may also find problems with how the child's digestive tract is working.
- Metal Detectors: This may be used to look for metal objects in the child's body, like coins.
- X-rays: X-rays of different parts of the child's body may be taken. These may include the neck, chest (lungs and heart), or abdomen. X-rays help caregivers look for the foreign body or signs of other problems. The child may need to have more than one x-ray.

## Treatment

Treatment will depend on the type and size of foreign body that the child has swallowed. Treatment also depends on how long and how far the foreign body is in the gastrointestinal (GI) tract. Most of the time, watchful waiting may be advised by the child's caregiver. Once the object is in his stomach, passing it out through the anus may be more likely. Passing out the object may take many days or weeks. The child may also have any of the following:

- Medicines: The child may be given sedatives and pain medicines to help him stay comfortable, calm, and relaxed. Antibiotic medicine may also be given to help treat or prevent an infection caused by germs called bacteria.
- Procedures: Removal of the object may be required if the object is stuck in the esophagus. This is also done if the object is sharp or pointed and may cause serious problems. Removing the object may be done using any of the following:

- Bougienage: Caregivers will insert a thin tube into the esophagus to widen it. They will then push the object into the stomach using another instrument. Bougienage is done if the object is smooth and blunt, and likely to be passed out the body. This may also be done if the object was swallowed within the past 24 hours.
- Endoscopy: A scope with a camera is passed through the child's mouth into his digestive tract. Caregivers look for the foreign body and remove it through the scope using different instruments. Objects may be grasped using forceps, or caught using a net. If the object to be taken out is sharp or pointed, it may be pulled out of the mouth. Caregivers may also treat other problems, like bleeding. Endoscopy may also be used to take out an object that can't go past the stomach.
- Foley catheter: Caregivers insert a catheter (rubber tube) into the mouth or nose till it goes past the object. With fluoroscopy (a special type of x-ray) as a guide, the balloon at the end of the catheter is filled, and gently pulled out. This may be done if the object is smooth or blunt, like a coin. A catheter may be used when the object was swallowed within the past 24 hours.

- Surgery: The child may need to have surgery if many objects were swallowed, or if the swallowed object was large. This may also be done to look for an injury or problem caused by the foreign body. Caregivers may also repair or treat the injury or problem during surgery.

## BURNS

From children washing up under a too-hot faucet to an accidental tipping of a coffee cup, burns are a potential hazard in every home. In fact, burns, particularly scalds from hot water and liquids, are some of the most common childhood accidents. Babies and young children are particularly susceptible - they're curious, small, and have sensitive skin that needs additional protection.

Though some minor burns aren't cause for concern and can be safely treated at home, other more serious burns require medical care. But taking some simple precautions to make the home safer can prevent many burns.

## Common Causes

The first step in helping to prevent the child from being burned is to understand the common causes of burns in children:

- Scalds, the number-one culprit (from steam, hot bath water, tipped-over coffee cups, cooking fluids, etc.)
- Contact with flames or hot objects (from the stove, fireplace, curling iron, etc.)
- Chemical burns (from swallowing things, such as drain cleaner or watch batteries, or spilling chemicals, like bleach, onto the skin)
- Electrical burns (from biting on electrical cords or sticking fingers or objects in electrical outlets, etc.)
- Overexposure to the sun

## Types

Burns are frequently categorized as first-, second-, or third-degree burns, depending upon how badly the skin is damaged. Each of the injuries above can cause any of these three types of burn. But both the type of burn and its cause will determine how the burn is treated. All burns ought to be treated rapidly to reduce the temperature of the burned area and reduce damage to the skin and underlying tissue (if the burn is severe).

First-degree burns, the mildest of the three, are limited to the top layer of skin:

- Signs and symptoms: These burns produce redness, pain, and minor swelling. The skin is dry without blisters.
- Healing time: Healing time is about 3 to 6 days; the superficial skin layer over the burn may peel off in 1 or 2 days.

Second-degree burns are more serious and involve the skin layers beneath the top layer:

- Signs and symptoms: These burns produce blisters, severe pain, and redness. The blisters sometimes break open and the area is wet looking with a bright pink to cherry red colour.
- Healing time: Healing time varies depending upon the severity of the burn.

Third-degree burns are the most serious type of burn and involve all the layers of the skin and underlying tissue:

- Signs and symptoms: The surface appears dry and can look waxy white, leathery, brown, or charred. There may be little or no pain or the area may feel numb at first due to nerve damage.
- Healing time: Healing time depends on the severity of the burn. Deep second- and third-degree burns (called full-thickness burns) will likely need to be treated with skin grafts, in which healthy skin is taken from another part of the body and surgically placed over the burn wound to help the area heal.

## Treatment

For First-Degree Burns:

- Remove the child from the heat source.
- Remove clothing from the burned area promptly.
- Run cool (not cold) water over the burned area (if water isn't available, any cold, drinkable fluid can be used) or hold a clean, cold compress on the burn for approximately 3 to 5 minutes (don't use ice, as it may cause the burn to take longer to heal).
- Don't apply butter, grease, powder, or any other remedies to the burn, as this increase the risk of infection.
- If the burned area is small, loosely cover it with a sterile gauze pad or bandage.
- Give the child acetaminophen or ibuprofen for pain.
- If the area affected is small (the size of a quarter or smaller), keep the area clean and continue to use cool compresses and a loose dressing over the next 24 hours. The parents can also apply antibiotic cream two to three times a day, though this isn't absolutely essential.

For Second- and Third-Degree Burns:

- Seek emergency medical care, then follow these steps till medical personnel arrive:
  - Keep the child lying down with the burned area elevated.
  - Follow the instructions for first-degree burns.
  - Remove all jewellery and clothing from around the burn (in case there's any swelling after the injury), except for clothing that's stuck to the skin. If the parents're having difficulty removing clothing, the parents may need to cut it off or wait till medical assistance arrives.

— Don't break any blisters.
— Apply cool water over the area for at least 3 to 5 minutes, then cover the area with a clean white cloth or sheet till help arrives.

For Flame Burns:

- Extinguish the flames by having the child roll on the ground.
- Cover him or her with a blanket or jacket.
- Remove smouldering clothing and any jewellery around the burned area.
- Call for medical assistance, then follow instructions for second- and third-degree burns.

For Electrical and Chemical Burns:

- Make sure the child is not in contact with the electrical source before touching him or her or the parents may also get shocked.
- Flush the burned area with lots of running water for 5 minutes or more. If the burned area is large, use a tub, shower, buckets of water, or a garden hose.
- Don't remove any of the child's clothing before the parents've begun flushing the burn with water. As the parents continue flushing the burn, the parents can then remove clothing from the burned area.
- If the burned area is small, flush for another 10 to 20 minutes, apply a sterile gauze pad or bandage, and call the child's physician.
- Chemical burns to the mouth or eyes require prompt medical assessment after thorough flushing with water.

Though both chemical and electrical burns might not always be visible, they can be serious due to potential damage to the child's internal organs. Symptoms may vary, depending upon the type and severity of the burn and what caused it and may include abdominal pain.

If the parents think the child may have swallowed a chemical substance or an object that could be unsafe (for example, a watch battery) first call poison control and then the emergency department. It is useful to know what chemical product the child has swallowed or has been exposed to. The parents may need to take it with the parents to the hospital. It's a good concept to have the number for poison control, in an easily accessible place, like on the refrigerator.

## DROWNING

From the time children are very young, they develop a curiosity about water that makes drowning a serious risk. People frequently think of pools, lakes and other large bodies of water as the primary sites of drowning danger for children. While many children drown in such circumstances, children under the age of one year are actually most likely to drown in bathtubs, buckets and toilets.

Drowning frequently occurs abruptly and without warning. Children can drown in less than 2 inches (5 centimeters) of water in a matter of just a few minutes. After the first year of life, males have a higher risk of drowning than females.

Parents, caregivers or others who see a child drowning should try to save the child without getting into the water. If it is not possible to reach the child from land, grab a towel, rope, life preserver or other sturdy object and swim out to the child.

Parents and other caretakers can take many steps to lower their child's risk of drowning. When children are young, empty water from a bathtub, pail or any other container promptly after use. Add childproof locks to toilet lids or latches to bathroom doors and store buckets in safe places.

As children grow older, there is an increased risk that they will drown in bodies of water like lakes, rivers, oceans and pools. The risk of drowning can be reduced - but not eliminated - by teaching children to swim and to follow other safety steps.

Families that don't have swimming pools are urged to delay installing a pool till a child is at least five years old. Households that already have pools should install a fence that is at least 4 feet (1.22 meters) high and that separates the pool from the rest of the house on all four sides. Preventing direct access to the swimming pool from the house may help prevent more than half of the pool-related drownings in young children. Other precautions can also lower the risk of a child drowning.

### Preventing Drowning

Parents can take many steps to lower their child's risk of drowning. Staying close to a child is amongst the most important of these steps. Parents are urged to remain within an arm's length of infants at all times when the young child is in water. This is known as "touch supervision." Supervising children around all sources of water is one of the most important prevention methods for drowning.

When children are young, empty water from a bathtub, pail or any other container immediately after use. Children can drown in less than 2 inches of water, so don't leave them unsupervised in or near any amount of water. This includes bathtubs, buckets, hot tubs and spas, wading pools, swimming pools, irrigation ditches and wells, fish ponds and fountains.

Toilets and buckets also present a drowning risk to children, as toddlers who reach into a toilet or bucket and fall in headfirst may not be strong enough to get themselves out. To prevent this, add childproof locks to toilet lids or latches to bathroom doors. In addition, store buckets in safe places and don't leave them outside, where they can accumulate water during storms.

As children grow older, the risk increases for drowning in bodies of water such as lakes, rivers, oceans and pools. The risk of drowning can be reduced - but not eliminated - by teaching children to swim. By age five, most children are developmentally ready to learn how to swim. However, even after they become proficient swimmers, five-year-olds are still too young to swim unsupervised. Never allow young children to swim without adult supervision.

While children learn to swim, teach them to limit the amount of time they spend in the water and to avoid deeper waters untiltill their technique has become proficient. It is important to remind children that swimming in lakes or oceans oftenfrequently requires more energy than swimming in pools. It is best to use caution when swimming in such bodies of water to avoid tiring while still far from the shore. Remind children to avoid waters that are not supervised by a lifeguard and to watch out for conditions such as changing currents, strong winds, sudden storms and rip tides. Teach children to swim with the current when caught in these conditions and gradually swim back to shore.

Teach children to enter a body of water feet-first during an initial entry into the water. Once the depth of the water is established, diving may be permitted. Diving headfirst into shallow bodies of water can cause permanent spinal cord damage if the head is injured. Don't allow children to play unsupervised around any bodies of water or to swim in any canal or near any fast-moving water.

All children should wear a life jacket when aboard any boat, regardless of distance to be traveled or the ability of the boaters to swim. Parents are urged to check the size and weight recommendations on these devices and to make sure each device fits snugly. For children younger than age five, choose a vest with a head support and a strap that fits between the legs. This will keep the child's head up and face out of the water. Air-filled swimming aids such as inner-tubes or water wings should not be used as personal flotation devices.

Exercise caution during other water-based activities, such as attending water parks. Don't use a park unless it is monitored by lifeguards and make sure children don't participate in any rides unless they meet the age, height, weight or health requirements.

Parents are urged to remain vigilant at all times regarding their child's safety around water. Most children who drown are in the care of their parents and are out of sight for less than five minutes, according to the CDC. Parents and caregivers also are urged to learn cardiopulmonary resuscitation (CPR) and other life-saving techniques from professionals so they can render care for their child, and other children, in an emergency.

As children grow older and become better swimmers, they may be allowed to swim unsupervised. Encourage older children to always swim with at least one other person. Also, remind children to avoid swimming or diving in areas indicated by off-limits signs.

A large percentage of drownings of older children involve alcohol. Teach older children not to use alcohol, especially before or during swimming.

## NURSING CARE OF INFANT AND CHILDREN WITH HIV/AIDS

Children living with HIV and AIDS will have special requirements that are different from those of adults. They are not able to get access to services and help themselves in the same way. Usually they depend on their mother or another caregiver. If they are very young, they will not understand the disease and the steps they have to take to stay healthy and to protect other people.

Most children with HIV and AIDS were infected as a result of mother - child transmission and their parents frequently become ill or die when the children are still very young. While all young orphans from poor families need a lot of different kinds of support, home-based care and child-care volunteers should make particularly sure that the medical requirements of children with HIV and AIDS are correctly addressed.

It is best for children to be looked after by those they know and make them feel safe. If possible, children with HIV and AIDS ought to be left in the care of their families and relatives. These relatives ought to be targeted for support. In some areas, there are hospices or homes for children who are ill or dying. Social workers should work with clinics, home-based care and child-care volunteers to identify children who would be better off in hospices.

Children with HIV and AIDS are just as subject to discrimination as adults but are much less able to fend for themselves. It is significant that every effort be made, by caregivers, teachers, healthcare providers, childcare committees and society leaders, to educate society members. People must fully understand, for instance, that an HIV-positive child can't spread HIV through sitting next to each other in class or playing together.

Most ill children are too small to care for themselves in any way. The caregiver has to be the major objective for support and training to make sure the child receives proper care. Childcare committees, local clinics or any person/organization having contact with caregivers should try and support the caregiver in anyway they can. This could include helping them find a support group, ensuring that they have applied for the right grants or sending them to special training.

## SPECIAL CARE CONSIDERATIONS FOR CHILDREN LIVING WITH HIV AND AIDS

### Antiretrovirals for Children

All HIV-positive children ought to be assessed at a clinic or hospital to see if they should start antiretroviral treatment (ATR). A syrup form of ART is available for children which is easier for them to take than tablets but ensuring compliance can be a major challenge. Children taking antiretrovirals need a lot of support and supervision to make sure they are taking the medicines correctly and as frequently as needed.

Children who suffer side effects after first going on antiretrovirals may not wish to continue on the medication. This is where they need an adult to encourage them to continue and/or make sure they return to the clinic on a regular basis (and if the side effects continue). As children grow, the dosage of the medications must be changed and this may need to happen several times per year. This underlines the importance of ensuring that the child gets to the clinic on a regular basis.

### Sanitation Considerations

Wash the hands before and after changing a nappy. Wear disposable gloves if there is blood in the faeces or urine, and if the parents have a rash or open cut on the hands. Place disposable nappies in a leak-proof container, like a plastic bag, and put it in a sealed rubbish bin.

Family-style eating is fine with everyone being served from a common serving dish. A child who is HIV-positive should use the same dishes, glasses, and eating utensils. The parents don't have to wash dishes and utensils separately. Wash all dishes in hot, soapy water. Clean and sterilize baby bottles as usual. Children who are HIV-positive should only use their own tooth brush and never share it.

Clothes that belong to a child who is HIV-positive can be washed with everyone else's clothes using ordinary washing powder or soap. If, however, the clothing has been soiled by blood, faeces, or vomit, wash items separately using 1/2 cup bleach.

## REFERENCES

Ashwill, Jean W. & Droske, Susan C. (1997). Nursing Care of Children, Philadelphia, PA: W. B. Saunders.

Ball, Jane & Binder, Ruth. (1999). Pediatric Nursing, 2nd ed., St. Louis, MO: Mosby.

Christensen, Barbara & Kockrow, Elaine. (1999). Foundations of Nursing, 3rd. ed., St. Louis, MO: Mosby.

James, Susan Rowan, Ashwill, Jean Weller, & Droske, Susan Colvert. (2002). Nursing Care of Children: Principles & Practice, 2nd ed., Philadelphia, PA: W. B. Saunders.

Leifer, Gloria. (1999). Thompson's Introduction to Maternity and Pediatric Nursing, 3rd ed., Philadelphia, PA: W. B. Saunders.

Marks, Margaret G. (1998). Broadribb's Introductory Pediatric Nursing, 5th ed., Philadelphia, PA: J. B. Lippincott.

Novak, Julie C. (1999). Novak: Ingalls & Salerno's Maternal & Child Health Nursing, 9th ed., St. Louis, MO: Mosby.

Opperman, C. & Cassandra, K. (1998). Contemporary Pediatric Nursing, St. Louis, MO: Mosby.

# 6

# Management of Behavioural & Social Problems in Children

All young children can be naughty, defiant and impulsive from time to time, which is perfectly normal. However, some children have extremely difficult and challenging behaviours that are outside the norm for their age.

The most common disruptive behaviour disorders include oppositional defiant disorder (ODD), conduct disorder (CD) and attention deficit hyperactivity disorder (ADHD). These three behavioural disorders share some common symptoms, so diagnosis can be difficult and time consuming. A child or adolescent may have two or even all three disorders at the same time. Other exacerbating factors can include emotional problems, mood disorders, family difficulties and substance abuse.

## Risk Factors

The causes of ODD, CD and ADHD are unknown but some of the risk factors include:

- Gender: boys are much more likely than girls to suffer from behavioural disorders. It is unclear if the cause is genetic or associated to socialisation experiences.
- Gestation and birth: difficult pregnancies, premature birth and low birth weight may contribute in some cases to the child's anti-social behaviour later in life.
- Temperament: children who are difficult to manage, temperamental or aggressive from an early age are more likely to develop behavioural disorders later in life.
- Family life: behavioural disorders are more likely in dysfunctional families. For instance, a child is at increased risk in families

where domestic violence, poverty, poor parenting skills or substance abuse are a problem.

- Learning difficulties: like problems with reading and writing.
- Intellectual disabilities: children with intellectual disabilities are twice as likely to have behavioural disorders.
- Brain activity: studies have shown that areas of the brain that control attention appear to be less active in children with ADHD.

## Diagnosis

Disruptive behavioural disorders are complicated and may include many different factors working in combination. For instance, a child who exhibits the delinquent behaviours of CD may also have ADHD, anxiety, depression, a drug use problem and a difficult home life. Diagnosis methods may include:

- Diagnosis by a specialist service, which may include a paediatrician, psychologist or child psychiatrist
- In-depth interviews with the parents, child and teachers
- Behaviour check lists or standardised questionnaires.

A diagnosis is made if the child's behaviour meets the criteria for disruptive behaviour disorders in the Diagnostic and Statistical Manual of Mental Disorders.

It is significant to rule out acute stressors that might be disrupting the child's behaviour. For instance, a sick parent or victimising by other children might be responsible for sudden changes in a child's typical behaviour and these factors have to be regarded initially.

## Treatment

Untreated children with behavioural disorders may grow up to be dysfunctional adults. In general, the earlier the intervention, the better the outcome is likely to be.

Treatment is usually multi-faceted and depends on the particular disorder and factors contributing to it, but may include:

- Parental education - for instance, teaching parents how to communicate with and manage their children.
- Functional family therapy - the entire family is helped to improve communication and problem-solving skills.

- Cognitive behavioural therapy - to help the child to control their thoughts and behaviour.
- Social training - the child is taught significant social skills, like how to have a conversation or play cooperatively with others.
- Anger management - the child is taught how to recognise the signs of their growing frustration and given a range of coping skills designed to defuse their anger and aggressive behaviour. Relaxation techniques and stress management skills are also taught.
- Support for associated problems - for instance, a child with a learning difficulty will benefit from professional support.
- Encouragement - many children with behavioural disorders experience repeated failures at school and in their interactions with others. Encouraging the child to excel in their particular talents (like sport) can help to build self-esteem.
- Medication - to help control impulsive behaviours.

## DISRUPTIVE BEHAVIOUR DISORDERS

Disruptive Behaviour Disorder is an expression used to describe a set of externalising negativistic behaviours that co-occur during childhood; and which are referred to collectively in the Diagnostic and Statistical Manual of Mental Disorders: Fourth Edition (DSM-IV) as: "Attention-Deficit and Disruptive Behaviour Disorders". There are three subgroups of externalising behaviours:

- Oppositional Defiant Disorder (ODD)
- Conduct Disorder (CD)
- Attention Deficit Hyperactivity Disorder (ADHD)

## OPPOSITIONAL DEFIANT DISORDER (ODD)

Oppositional Defiant Disorder (ODD) consists of a pattern of negativistic, hostile, and defiant behaviour lasting at least 6 months, during which four (or more) of the following behaviours are present:

- Frequently loses temper
- Frequently argues with adults
- Frequently dynamically defies or refuses to comply with adults' requests or rules
- Frequently deliberately annoys people

- Frequently blames others for his or her mistakes or misbehaviour
- Is frequently touchy or easily annoyed by others
- Is frequently angry and resentful
- Is frequently spiteful or vindictive

Each of the above is only regarded diagnostic if the behaviour occurs more regularly than is typically observed in children of comparable age and developmental level and if the behaviour causes clinically significant impairment in social, academic, or occupational functioning.

Oppositional Defiant disorder is not diagnosed if the behaviours occur exclusively during the course of a Psychotic or Mood Disorder or if Conduct Disorder is diagnosed.

## CONDUCT DISORDER

The DSM-IV categorises conduct disorder behaviours into four major groupings: (a) aggressive conduct that causes or threatens physical harm to other people or animals, (b) non- aggressive conduct that causes property loss or damage, (c) deceitfulness or theft, and (d) serious violations of rules. Conduct Disorder consists of a repetitive and persistent pattern of behaviours in which the fundamental rights of others or major age-appropriate norms or rules of society are violated. Typically there would have been three or more of the following behaviours in the past 12 months, with at least one in the past 6 months:

- Frequently bullies, threatens, or intimidates others
- Frequently starts physical fights
- Has used a weapon that can cause serious physical harm to others (e.g., a bat, brick, broken bottle, knife, gun)
- Has been physically cruel to people
- Has been physically cruel to animals
- Has stolen while confronting a victim (e.g., mugging, purse snatching, extortion, armed robbery)
- Has forced someone into sexual activity
- Has deliberately engaged in fire setting with the intention of causing serious damage
- Has deliberately destroyed others' property (other than by fire setting)

- Has broken into someone else's house, building, or car
- frequently lies to obtain goods or favours or to avoid obligations (i.e., "cons" others)
- Has stolen items of nontrivial value without confronting a victim (e.g., shoplifting, but without breaking and entering; forgery)
- Frequently stays out at night in spite of parental prohibitions, beginning before age 13 years.
- Has run away from home overnight at least twice while living in parental or parental surrogate home (or once without returning for a lengthy period).
- Is frequently truant from school, beginning before age 13 years.

## Subtypes of Conduct Disorder

There are two subtypes of conduct disorder outlined in DSM-IV, and their diagnosis differs primarily as per the nature of the presenting problems and the course of their development.

The first, childhood-onset type, is defined by the onset of one criterion characteristic of conduct disorder before age 10. Children with childhood-onset conduct disorder are usually male, and regularly display physical aggression; they usually have disturbed peer relationships, and may have had oppositional defiant disorder during early childhood. These children usually meet the full criteria for conduct disorder before puberty, they are more likely to have persistent conduct disorder, and are more likely to develop adult antisocial personality disorder than those with the adolescent-onset type.

The second, the adolescent-onset type, is defined by the absence of conduct disorder prior to age 10. As compared to individuals with the childhood-onset type, they are less likely to display aggressive behaviours. These individuals tend to have more normal peer relationships, and are less likely to have persistent conduct disorders or to develop adult antisocial personality disorder. The ratio of males to females is also lower than for the childhood-onset type.

## Severity of Symptoms

Conduct disorder is classified as "mild" if there are few, if any, conduct problems in excess of those needed for diagnosis and if these cause only minor harm to others (e.g., lying, truancy and breaking parental rules). A classification of "moderate" is applied when the number of conduct problems and effect on others are intermediate between "mild" and "severe". The "severe" classification is justified when many conduct problems exist which are in excess of those needed for diagnosis, or the conduct problems cause considerable harm to others or property (e.g., rape, assault, mugging, breaking and entering).

### Co-morbidities and Associated Disorders

Children with conduct disorder are part of a population within which there are higher incidences of a number of disorders than in a normal population. The literature abounds with studies indicating the comorbid relationships between Attention Deficit Hyperactivity Disorder, Conduct Disorder, Oppositional Defiant Disorder, Learning Difficulties, Mood Disorders, Depressive symptoms, Anxiety Disorders, Communication Disorders, and Tourettes Disorder.. A high level of co-morbidity (almost 95%) was found amongst 236 ADHD children (aged 6-16 yrs) with conduct disorder, ODD and other related categories (Bird, Gould, & Staghezza Jaramillo, 1994). In an 8 year follow-up study, Barklay and colleagues (1990) found that 80% of the children with ADHD were still hyperactive as adolescents and that 60% of them had developed Oppositional Defiant or Conduct Disorder.

### Prevalence of Conduct Disorder

The incidence of the disorder is thought to vary demographically, with some areas being worse than others. Because prevalence estimates are based primarily upon referral rates, and because many children and adolescents are never referred for mental health services, the actual incidences may well be higher.

## CAUSES OF CONDUCT DISORDER

There is evidence from research into causes of conduct disorders that indicates that several biological and environmental factors may contribute to the development of the disorder.

Neurological Dysregulation: The high co-morbidity rate of Conduct Disorder with ADHD, Tourettes syndrome and other disorders known to be because of neurological dysregulation suggests that Conduct Disorder may be a co-manifestation of the same underlying dysregulation. Though there are no studies to our knowledge, which have directly investigated the neurological basis for conduct disorder, there is ample clinical evidence indicating that when treating ADHD with Neurotherapy, and Nutrient supplementation, Conduct Disorder abates. It appears that Neurotherapy may address the underlying dysregulation and facilitate clinical treatment using cognitive and behavioural interventions. More research is required in this area to determine whether Neurotherapy is directly responsible for this abatement or whether the resultant improvement in attention, and reduction in hyperactivity promotes better self image which in turn improves behaviour.

Child Biological Factors: Considerable research has been carried out into the role of child temperament, the tendency to respond in predictable ways to events, as a predictor of conduct problems. Aspects of the personality like activity levels displayed by a child, emotional responsiveness, quality of mood and social adaptability are part of his or her temperament. Longitudinal studies have found that though there is a relationship between early patterns of temperament, and adaptation during adulthood, the longer the time span the weaker this relationship becomes.

A more significant determinant of whether or not temperamental qualities persist has been shown to be the manner in which parents respond to their children. "Difficult" infants have been shown to be particularly likely to display behaviour problems later in life if their parents are impatient, inconsistent, and demanding.

On the other hand "difficult" infants, whose parents give them time to adapt to new experiences, learn to master new situations effectively. In a favourable family context a "difficult" infant is not at risk of displaying disruptive behaviour disorder at 4 years old.

Cognitions may also influence the development of conduct disorder. Children with conduct disorder have been found to misinterpret or distort social cues during interactions with peers. For instance, a neutral situation may be construed as having hostile intent.

Further, children who are aggressive have been shown to seek fewer cues or facts when interpreting the intent of others. Children with conduct disorder experience deficits in social problem solving skills. As a result they generate fewer alternate solutions to social problems, seek less information, see problems as having a hostile basis, and anticipate fewer consequences than children who don't have a conduct disorder.

School-Related Factors: A bidirectional relationship exists between academic performance and conduct disorder. Regularly children with conduct disorder exhibit low intellectual functioning and low academic achievement from the outset of their school years. Particularly, reading disabilities have been linked with this disorder, with one study finding that children with conduct disorder were at a reading level 28 months behind normal peers.

In addition, delinquency rates and academic performance have been shown to be associated with characteristics of the school setting itself. Such factors as physical attributes of the school, teacher availability, teacher use of praise, the quantity of emphasis placed on personal duty, emphasis on academic work, and the student teacher ratio have been implicated.

Parent Psychological Factors: It is known that a child's risk of developing conduct disorder is increased in the event of parent psychopathology. Maternal depression, paternal alcoholism and/or criminalism and antisocial behaviour in either parent have been specially linked to the disorder.

There are two views as to why maternal depression has this effect. The first considers that mothers who are depressed misperceive their child's behaviour as maladjusted or inappropriate. The second considers the influence depression can have on the way a parent reacts toward misbehaviour. Depressed mothers have been shown to direct a higher number of commands and criticisms towards their children, who in turn respond with increased noncompliance and deviant child behaviour. Webster-Stratton and Dahl proposed that depressed and irritable mothers indirectly cause behaviour problems in their children through inconsistent limit setting, emotional unavailability, and reinforcement of inappropriate behaviours through negative attention.

Familial Contributions: The inter-parental conflicts surrounding divorce have been linked with the development of conduct disorder. However, it has been noted that though some single parents and their children become chronically depressed and report increased stress levels after separation, others do comparatively well. Forgatch proposed that for some single parents, the events surrounding separation and divorce set off a period of increased depression and irritability which leads to loss of support and friendship, setting in place the risk of more irritability, ineffective discipline, and poor problem solving outcomes. The ineffective problem solving can result in more depression, while the increase in irritable behaviour may simultaneously lead the child to become antisocial.

More detailed researches into the effects of parental separation and divorce on child behaviour have revealed that the intensity of conflict and discord between the parents, instead of divorce itself, is the significant factor. Children of divorced parents whose homes are free from conflict have been found to be less likely to have problems than children whose parents remained together but engaged in a great deal of conflict, or those who continued to have conflict after divorce. Webster noted that half of all those children referred to their clinic with conduct problems were from families with a history of marital spouse abuse and violence.

In addition to the effect of marital conflict on the child, conflict can also regulate parenting behaviours. Marital conflict has been linked with inconsistent parenting, higher levels of punishment with a concurrent reduction in reasoning and rewards, as well as with parents taking a negative perception of their child's adaptation.

Family Adversity and Insularity: Life stressors like poverty, unemployment, overcrowding, and ill health are known to have an adverse effect on parenting and to be consequently associated with the development of conduct disorder. The presence of major life stressors in the lives of families with conduct disordered children has been found to be two to four times greater than in other families.

Mothers' perception of the availability of supportive and social contact has also been implicated in child contact disorder. Mothers who don't believe supportive social contact is available are termed "insular" and have been found to use more aversive consequences with their children than non-insular mothers.

Parent Child Interactions: Research has suggested that parents of children with conduct disorder regularly lack several significant parenting skills. Parents have been reported to be more violent and critical in their use of discipline, more inconsistent, erratic, and permissive, less likely to monitor their children, as well as more likely to punish pro-social behaviours and to reinforce negative behaviours. A coercive process is set in motion during which a child escapes or avoids being criticised by his or her parents through producing an increased number of negative behaviours. These behaviours lead to increasingly aversive parental reactions which serve to reinforce the negative behaviours.

Differences in affect have also been noted in conduct disordered children. Generally their affect is less positive, they appear to be depressed, and are less reinforcing to their parents. These attributes can set the scene for the cycle of aversive interactions between parents and children.

## TREATMENT

A number of interventions have been identified which are helpful in reducing the prevalence and incidence of conduct disorder. Interventions consist of prevention and treatment, though these shouldn't be regarded as separate entities. Prevention addresses the onset of the disorder, though the child has not manifested the disorder, and treatment addresses reduction of the severity of the disorder. In mainstream Psychology, prevention and treatment for Conduct Disorder primarily focuses on skill development, not only for the child but for others involved with the child, including the family and the school environments.

As previously discussed there may be clinical advantages in applying nutritional supplementation and Neurotherapy where appropriate with Conduct Disorder clients, if the client appears to respond to this form of neurological intervention, followed by cognitive and behavioural intervention. The following paragraphs considers three interventions, that assist in preventing and treating conduct disorder; child training, family training, and school and society interactions.

Child Training: Child training involves the teaching of new skills to facilitate the child's growth, development and adaptive functioning. Research indicates that as a means of preventing child conduct disorder there is a need for skill development in the area of child competence. Competence refers to the ability for the child to negotiate the course of development including effective interactions with others, successful completion of developmental tasks and contacts with the environment, and use of approaches that increase adaptive functioning. It has been found that facilitating the development of competence in children is helpful as a preventative measure for children prior to manifestation of the disorder instead of as a treatment.

Additionally, treatment interventions have been developed to focus on altering the child's cognitive processes. This includes teaching the child problem solving skills, self control facilitated by self statements and developing prosocial instead of antisocial behaviours. Prosocial skills are developed through the teaching of appropriate play skills, development of friendships and conversational skills. The social development of children provides them with the essential skills to interact positively in their environment. A child's development of cognitive skills provides a sound basis from which to proceed. However, cognitive development shouldn't be considered in isolation, but as part of a system, which highlights the need to include the family in the training process.

Family Intervention: A child's family system, has a significant role in the prevention and treatment of conduct disorder. The child needs to be regarded as a component of a system, instead of as a single entity. Research supports the idea that parents of conduct disordered children have underlying deficits in certain fundamental parenting skills. The development of effective parenting skills has been regarded as the primary mechanism for change in child conduct disorder, through the reduction of the severity, duration and manifestation of the disorder.

A number of parent training programs have been developed to increase parenting skills. Research indicates that the parent training programs have been positive, indicating significant changes in parents' and children's behaviour and parental perception of child adaptation. Research suggests that parents who have participated in parent training programs are successful in reducing their child's level of aggression by 20 - 60 %.

Several training programs have been developed, which focus on increasing parents' skills in managing their child's behaviour and facilitating social skills development. The skills focused on, include parents learning to assist in administration of appropriate reinforcement and disciplinary techniques, effective communication with the child and problem solving and negotiation strategies.

A further constituent of parental training incorporates behavioural management. This involves rendering the family with simple and effective strategies including behavioural contracting, contingency management, and the ability to facilitate generalisation and maintenance of their new skills, thus encouraging parents' positive interaction with their child.

However, though these interventions assist parents in developing effective parenting skills, a number of families require extra support. There are several characteristics within the family system that can have an impact on parents' ability to cope. This includes depression, life stress and marital distress. Research suggests that family characteristics are linked with fewer treatment gains in parent training programs. As indicated by Webster-Stratton and Dahl (1995), several programs have expanded upon the standard parent training treatment. These programs have incorporated parents' cognitive, psychological, and marital or social adaptation. Through addressing the parent's own issues it assists their ability to manage and interact positively with the child.

## MENTALLY CHALLENGED CHILDREN

One of the strongest factors is hereditary. Besides this there are a number of environmental factors that contribute to mental arrest. Most common of which is brain damage, malnutrition or infection during pregnancy or even an excessive intake of drugs and RH incompatibility. Whatsoever the cause, if the handicap is very severe, the total development of the child gets affected - physical, social and emotional along with mental. Some of these children can't perform the simplest of tasks that we all seem to take for granted. Simple things such as walking straight, eating or toilet training. A great quantity of patience and tolerance is needed to supervise and handle such a child.

The earlier the problem is detected the better it is for the parents and the child. Sometimes parents try to hide the fact till it becomes evident to all, and by then it is too late to get timely help. There are plenty of child counselling centres and special schools around to render the perfect environment to aid in the development of the child. But if these facilities are not utilized, a mentally deficient child will definitely develop severe social and emotional problems as well.

Parents should try to accept the fact that their child is mentally challenged and help him or her grow to the full potential that he or she is capable of. Some people try for a miraculous cure and expend a lot of time and energy in search of a divine elixir. Although such an attitude is understandable, it doesn't show any results. That time will be better spent in admitting the child to a special school or sheltered institution where he can get professional help.

Such schools teach the child how to survive and progress in our world. Special skills are taught to them to help them make good use of their time and lives. Each child is given a task that suits his or her mental growth. Sensory training and perceptual knowledge is stressed on and children are taught utilitarian tasks that will help the child to be more independent. This is generally taught through drill and repetition over a period of years.

Besides schools, parents and family members at home also must render a secure environment for the development of the abilities and interests of the mentally retarded. Parents shouldn't feel awkward and should help their child to socialise with family members, relatives and friends. Subnormal children need more love and affection than the normal child does or they tend to get frustrated. They might not be able to express their needs. So it is up to the parents to anticipate what they want and give them all the love and strength that they require to help them develop to their full potential.

India is holding nearly 1/6th of the world population and a large number of them are living beneath the poverty level. They have very limited access to the fundamental education, primary health facilities and employment opportunities.

Unfortunately, there are a number of children in these poor localities whose mental level is not at par with the other children. In real terms, they are mentally challenged up somewhat. Because of poverty and lack of resources, these children fail to receive due attention of their families and friends. They don't get sufficient support and motivation from the society to have access to fundamental education and develop their skills to become self reliant. They are being treated as a big burden for the family and besides, for the rest of the world. They don't get due affection, recreation and parental care. As a result, countless children with special learning requirements are not only deprived of fundamental education and healthcare but also live an isolated life even in their own house. Volunteers with their sincere efforts make tremendous impact on mentally challenged children by giving them fundamental education and skill development tips to improve their quality of life. Besides, Volunteers pay due attention towards the children's individual behaviour, their health, food, care and small requirements. Volunteers with their active participation are able to motivate their parents to send the children to schools on a regular basis. Besides, they motivate the society to be more sympathetic towards these children and support them by giving encouragement and due regards in the society.

## PHYSICALLY CHALLENGED CHILDREN

Children who are physically challenged need special care to overcome or reduce their disability. Parenting an exceptional child is distinctive in degree and intensity instead of in kind. Like all children exceptional children need love, care, counselling and protection from parents. The birth of an exceptional child adds a situation crisis, one that results from an unanticipated, traumatic event beyond parents control. Parents progress through six emotional stages upon discovering their child's exceptionality viz. disbelief, guilt, rejection, shame, denial and a feeling of helplessness upon discovering their child's exceptionality.

Parents must essentially learn to manipulate the environment for their children's benefit protecting them from social forces that conflict with their parenting philosophy and objectives. If the parents are supportive and encouraging and convey to the child that they are with them, then with patience optimism and understanding much of the restrictions placed by the impairment can be overcome. In such an environment the child will develop positive feelings about himself. Moreover parents who receive education through therapeutic programs, counselling or training courses help in caring a disabled child and in reducing his degree of disability.

Infants need to learn how to focus and attend to things apart from themselves. That involves coordinating what a baby sees with what he hears; naturally, he wants to look toward the voice of Mommy. But that might require turning his head, which can be hard for a child with low muscle tone or a weakness or rigidity on one side. So learning to focus and pay attention is the first challenge.

Then, babies must learn to engage another person. It's significant not only to look and listen, but to respond with great big smiles and enticing glances to woo parents into a loving relationship. That can be even more difficult for a child who can not turn, move easily, or reach up with her arms in efforts to get a hug, or move her face into big smiles.

Next, babies must learn to act purposefully. This involves exchanging emotional expressions and interactions - taking toys that are offered and handing them back, all while making gleeful sounds. But that is difficult too, if the parents can not move the arms or grasp something offered to the parents.

Children must also be able to perform a sequence of activities in order to problem-solve - for instance, taking Mommy by the hand, walking her to the toy area, pointing to the toy the parents want, and climbing up on Mommy's lap to reach it. Obviously, if the parents have severe motor problems, all those actions are difficult.

Using concepts creatively is another skill children must master. To do this, they have to be able to engage in pretend play, which might include picking up the doll, talking to it, and organizing a tea party. All of this involves complicated motor behaviour.

Finally, children need to learn to connect concepts. Some of the ways children do this are by talking with one another and by joining in games like musical chairs or ring around the rosy. Obviously, it's difficult to get involved in such activities when the parents have speech and motor difficulties.

The parents can see that motor skills play a big part in the overall development of children and that the challenges for a child with motor delays go way beyond having a hard time writing, running, and jumping.

## CHILD GUIDANCE CLINICS

The Department of Child and Adolescent Psychiatry (DCAP) provides psychological, psychiatric and educational services for children and adolescents up to 19 years of age. The vast majority of children and adolescents seen by the department don't suffer from mental illness. Most have emotional and behavioural problem that needs professional help.

The department runs a Child Guidance Clinic (CGC) located at Health Promotion Board and at Clinic B, IMH. There is also a Child and Adolescent Inpatient Unit at IMH/WH for inpatients. In addition, it runs the Children's One-Stop Psycho-Educational Services (COPES) at CGC.

Child Guidance Clinics render evaluation and treatment for the following:

- Behavioural problems e.g. lying, stealing, aggressiveness, destructiveness, disobedience, over activity
- Learning disabilities
- Emotional problem e.g. depression, school refusal, fears
- Adjustment reactions e.g. school related problem, grief
- Development disorder e.g. autism, bedwetting and soiling
- Intellectual deficit
- Psychosomatic disorders
- Bizarre and abnormal behaviours
- Relationship (including parent-child, sibling and marital) problem.
- Sociolegal issues and problem e.g. child custody evaluation, sexual offences, child abuse and head injuries.
- Other e.g. eating and sleep disorders, sexual problems in adolescence, tics (movement disorder) and stress reaction

## TREATMENT

Treatment is designed to meet each child's requirements. Treatment method used at our clinic include:

- Medical treatment
- Personal psychotherapy
- Family and martial therapy
- Behavioural/Cognitive therapy
- Occupational therapy
- Group therapy
- Play therapy
- Social case work

The child, being always dependent, has to be provided for by its parents and the family, the society and-the State. Considering the size of the-population involved and the nature and complexness of the problem, the total duty of welfare has to be borne cumulatively by the family, the regional society, and the State at three different levels. The problem of survival and the high incidence of infant mortality and birthrate has been dealt with in the chapter on Health. However, certain aspects of the problem of health, growth and care of the child need the attention of social welfare, agencies.

In a country where poverty is extensive, there is need to supplement the diet of children. Effective ways have to be devised by the State and private agencies to see that the essential nourishment is received at least by under-nourished children in schools and in established institutions. To augment State resources, an effort ought to be made by each local society to assist educational institutions and child welfare organizations in supplementing the diet of the child in some way.

At present, skimmed milk powder, cases of baby foods, semolina, vitamin tablets, pabulum cereals, codliver oil, etc., are received as gifts from several sources. Efforts to organise collections in kind at the society level could be supplemented by grants-in-aid from charity trusts and local self-governing bodies. It is desirable that State organizations, the Red Cross, the Indian Council of Child Welfare and other significant national and State organizations for child welfare should co-ordinate their efforts both for the collection and distribution of supplementary foods for children. The five most appropriate agencies for the distribution of free foods to children at the society level are (1) milk centres (2) maternity and child welfare centres (3) society centres (4) day nurseries and schools, and (5) play centres.

Feeble-mindedness: The attention of the educational authorities is naturally concentrated in the early stages on formal education. The problem of feeblemindedness is gradually beginning to receive the attention of psychologists and educationists in the country. Uptil now there are no adequate institutions in the country for the care and treatment of feeble-minded children.

A beginning has been made in dealing with this problem by the Society for the care, treatment, and training of children in need of special care. A few pilot projects in selected areas could be developed by specialised agencies for child welfare. One of the major handicaps in this respect is the absence of a enough number of trained psychologists and psychiatrists and teachers specifically trained to deal with mentally backward children. Provision ought to be made for training personnel as early as possible.

Child Guidance Clinics: The first child guidance clinic was organised in India in 1936. Since then a small number of child guidance clinics have been brought into existence in some of the larger cities. It is desirable that at least one child guidance clinic ought to be brought into existence in every State and, wherever possible, such clinics ought to be organised by municipalities. The Organization of this significant service is also likely to be handicapped because of want of psychiatrists and child psychologists. It is necessary to train a number of psychologists and case, workers in the schools of social work in order to render trained personnel for dealing with problem children.

Creches: A significant service which has already made considerable headway in India for the welfare of children is the Organization of creches, day nurseries and other types of pre-schools. In large factories in major cities, already a number of creches are organised with a reasonable standard of efficiency in the interest for children whose mothers work in the factories. In 1951, Bombay had 177 creches with about 3,000 children, Madras had 93 with about 2,334 children, Bihar had 26 with 796 children, Madhya Pradesh had 16 with 360 children and Uttar Pradesh had 7 with 126 children.

These figures reveal that only a very small percentage of children of working mothers take advantage of these creches, specifically because it is the tradition in India for children to be looked after by other women members of the family. As it is now compulsory under the Factories Act of 1948 to render a creche in factories employing 250 or more women special efforts may be made by factory owners to induce mothers to send their children to the creches.

Play Activities: Play is a vital need in the life of the child; and its playlife in the home, school and society environments consists of playthings, companionship, and playground activities. Local self-governing bodies as well as the society should render playspace for children either as a reserved part of a society playground, or as a separate playground equipped with appropriate accessories for play. Only a small number of fairly well- equipped playgrounds are in existence in the country; and their number needs to be very considerably increased in urban as well as rural areas. Proper maintenance and management of playgrounds are necessary in order to render essential guidance, supervision, and protection to children during play hours. Such a playground service could be provided by voluntary welfare agencies and the parentsth and students' organizations.

Children's Centre: In order to extend the scope of children's recreations, the programmes for children's centres are now being expanded so that they can be equipped with playgrounds, indoor space for a children's library, a dramatic hall, and facilities for developing child arts and handicrafts. Such centres may also render a case work service where it is not possible to organise a child guidance clinic.

Handicapped Children: One of the most difficult problems which deserves urgent consideration is the problem of lone, orphaned, neglected, deserted and destitute children. It is essential to develop special institutions, children's villages, boys' towns and similar organizations where a large number of such children could be given protection, shelter, care, education and training until they are rehabilitated and can function in a usual way. At present, such institutions are mainly organised by private agencies, and particularly by children's aid societies. Most of these institutions deal with a very small number of children, and it is desirable to start a number of pilot projects where a large number of children could be brought together under the care of specialised social welfare agencies in the several States.

The practice of adoption has existed in India for centuries. Such religious adoptions are not legally controlled. Also,, this benefit is invariably given to the boy. In some cases the orphaned child is institutionalised, or becomes a beggar, or becomes a victim of illegal trafficking and exploitation. Orphanages exist all over the country, both in urban and rural areas. The need to ensure registration, supervision and control of these institutions is now realised, and legislation and machinery of enforcement have to be devised to protect children in institutions organised by private agencies. Such institutions, with the support of the Government, ought to be able to render a reasonable opportunity for growth, development and rehabilitation of all the inmates.

Juvenile Delinquency: The complexities of the problem of delinquency and the deficiency of resources, institutions, and personnel have come in the way of a study of the nature and extent of the problem. At present, only a small number of delinquent children are dealt with, and the treatment given to them doesn't render for full rehabilitation. The problem of delinquency is extensive due to the prevailing normal conditions in which children are brought up. Poverty, neglect, slum life and frustration may lead to acts of delinquency. Case treatment frequently reveals the delinquency of the parent, experience of cruelty at home, and encouragement of delinquent acts by elders.

In some States progressive legislation for dealing with delinquency already exists in others, no legislation has yet been enacted. The Ministry of Education has drafted model legislation for the guidance of States. Most of the Children's Acts deal with neglected, dependent and destitute children, difficult, uncontrollable and delinquent children and victimised and exploited children. In some cases the provisions of the Children's Act are in conflict with Wards and Guardians Acts. All existing legislation and treatment ought to be reviewed from the standpoint of a more complete approach towards the problem.

The weakest link in the treatment of the problem is the absence of one appropriate agency for the enforcement of the legislation, the absence of an adequate police force, and deficiency of court facilities, children's institutions, and probation officers. It is essential to set up juvenile aid committees in cities, consisting of a small number of selected and specifically trained police officials who will examine cases of delinquents, and deal with cases of minor delinquencies without reference to courts.

The deficiency of existing certified schools' and fit-persons institutions is well known, and in order to render the right conditions, a beginning has been made in some States to create children's villages, boys' towns and other institutions with proper conditions of rehabilitation. Pilot projects for this purpose are contemplated in certain States where the incidence of delinquency is high. Institutions such as juvenile reformatories exist in the country, and these need to be adapted and re-organised to suit the present objectives. The practice of rendering even temporary habitation and shelter to juveniles in correctional institutions where adult under-trials and prisoners live ought to be discontinued.

The normal improvement of child welfare services in India calls for greater coordination and better leadership for the several hundred child welfare organizations that exist in India. The child welfare movement, under the guidance of the Indian Council for Child Welfare needs to be encouraged and strengthened; and it ought to be made more representative of children's organizations in the country.

There ought to be a strong national headquarters to carry out the objectives of the movement, and maintain and improve standards of child welfare. It is proposed to create a national centre of child welfare in a central place, with similar organizations in some of the States. The national centre will become the experimental station, training centre, seat of pilot projects and clearing house for information and material on child welfare.

Children's Organizations: Although relatively small in size, organizations for children have come into existence in different parts of India for rendering recreation for children. The Balkan-ji-Bari is a developing Organization and its major value lies in bringing together children from all over India in camps and national festivals. The Bachon-ki-Biradari and Kishore Dal are similar organizations in the north. Such organizations deserve the support of local self-governing bodies and child welfare agencies. The junior sections of the Boy Scouts and Girl Guides organizations have been long engaged in giving valuable training to children outside the educational institutions. These organizations help to develop children for a fitting role in the the parentsth movement.

## REFERENCES

Ashwill, Jean W. & Droske, Susan C. (1997). Nursing Care of Children, Philadelphia, PA: W. B. Saunders.

Ball, Jane & Binder, Ruth. (1999). Pediatric Nursing, 2nd ed., St. Louis, MO: Mosby.

Christensen, Barbara & Kockrow, Elaine. (1999). Foundations of Nursing, 3rd. ed., St. Louis, MO: Mosby.

Leifer, Gloria. (1999). Thompson's Introduction to Maternity and Pediatric Nursing, 3rd ed., Philadelphia, PA: W. B. Saunders.

Marks, Margaret G. (1998). Broadribb's Introductory Pediatric Nursing, 5th ed., Philadelphia, PA: J. B. Lippincott.

Novak, Julie C. (1999). Novak: Ingalls & Salerno's Maternal & Child Health Nursing, 9th ed., St. Louis, MO: Mosby.

Opperman, C. & Cassandra, K. (1998). Contemporary Pediatric Nursing, St. Louis, MO: Mosby.

Pilliterri, Adele. (2003). Maternal and Child Health Nursing, 4th ed., Philadelphia, PA: J. B. Lippincott.

Pilliterri, Adele. (1999). Maternal and Child Health Nursing, 3rd ed., Philadelphia, PA: J. B. Lippincott.

Pilliterri, Adele. (1999). Children's Health Nursing: Care of the Child and Family, 1st ed., Philadelphia, PA: J. B. Lippincott.

Schulte, Elizabeth B., Price, Debra L., & Gwin, Julie F. (2001). Thompson's Pediatric Nursing, 8th ed., Philadelphia, PA: W. B. Saunders.

White, Lois. (2002) Basic Nursing Foundations of Skills and Concepts, Albany, NY: Delmar Publishing.

Wong, Donna L. (1997). Whaley & Wong's Essentials of Pediatric Nursing, 5th ed., St. Louis, MO: Mosby.

Wong, Donna L., Hockenberry-Eaton, Marilyn, Wilson, David, Winkelstien, Marilyn, Schwartz, Patricia. (2001). Whaley & Wong's Essentials of Pediatric Nursing, 6th ed., St. Louis, MO: Mosby.

Wong, Donna L., Hockenberry-Eaton, Marilyn, Wilson, David, Winkelstien, Marilyn, Attmann, Elizabeth, & DiVito-Thomas,

Pamela A. (1999). Nursing Care of Infants and Children, 6th ed., St. Louis, MO: Mosby.

Wong, Donna L., Perry, Shannon E., & Hockenberry, Marilyn J. (2002). Maternal Child Nursing Care, 2nd ed., St. Louis, MO: Mosby.

# Bibliography


Algranati PS. Effect of developmental status on the approach to physical examination. Pediatr Clin North Am 1998; 45(1): 1-23.

Algranati PS. The pediatric patient: an approach to history and physical examination. Baltimore: Williams & Wilkins; 1992.

Ashwill, Jean W. & Droske, Susan C. (1997). Nursing Care of Children, Philadelphia, PA: W. B. Saunders.

Ball, Jane & Binder, Ruth. (1999). Pediatric Nursing, 2nd ed., St. Louis, MO: Mosby.

Behrman R, Vaughan W. Nelson's textbook of pediatrics, 16th edn. St. Louis: WB Saunders; 1999.

Boynton R. Manual of ambulatory pediatrics, 4th edn. Philadelphia: Lippincott; 1998.

Brundige KJ. Preparing pediatric nurse practitioners for roles in specialty practice. J Pediatr Health Care 1997; 11(4):198-200.

Burns C. Pediatric primary care: a handbook for nurse practitioners, 2nd edn. London: WB Saunders; 2000.

Callender D. Pediatric practice guidelines: implications for nurse practitioners. J Pediatr Health Care 1999;

Christensen, Barbara & Kockrow, Elaine. (1999). Foundations of Nursing, 3rd. ed., St. Louis, MO: Mosby.

Coupey SM. Interviewing adolescents. Pediatr Clin North Am 1997; 44(6):1349-1364.

Ehram W, Matson S. Approach to assessing adolescents on serious or sensitive issues. Pediatr Clin North Am 1998; 45(1):189-204.

Elster A, Levenberg P. Integrating comprehensive adolescent preventive services into routine medical care. Pediatr Clin North Am 1997; 44(6):1365-1377.

Engel J. Pocket guide to pediatric assessment, 3rd edn. St. Louis: Mosby; 1997.

Gaedeke MK. Advanced practice nursing in pediatric acute care. Crit Care Nurs Clin North Am 1995; 7(1):61-70.

Gill D, O'Brien N. Paediatric clinical examination, 3rd edn. London: Churchill Livingstone; 1998.

Ginsburg K. Guiding adolescents away from violence. Contemp Pediatr 1997; Goldenring JM, Cohen E. Getting into adolescent heads. Contemp Pediatr 1989; 5:75-90.

Hillard P. Preserving confidentiality in adolescent gynecology. Contemp Pediatr 1997; 14(6):71-92.

James, Susan Rowan, Ashwill, Jean Weller, & Droske, Susan Colvert. (2002). Nursing Care of Children: Principles & Practice, 2nd ed., Philadelphia, PA: W. B. Saunders.

Jarvis C. Physical examination and health assessment, 2nd edn. Philadelphia: WB Saunders; 1996.

Knight J. Adolescent substance use: screening, assessment, and intervention. Contemp Pediatr 1997; 14(4):45-72.

Leifer, Gloria. (1999). Thompson's Introduction to Maternity and Pediatric Nursing, 3rd ed., Philadelphia, PA: W. B. Saunders.

MacGregor J. Introduction to the anatomy and physiology of children. London: Routledge; 2000.

Marks, Margaret G. (1998). Broadribb's Introductory Pediatric Nursing, 5th ed., Philadelphia, PA: J. B. Lippincott.

Neinstein LS. Adolescent health care, 3rd edn. London: Williams & Wilkins; 1996.

Nicholson D, Ayers H. Adolescent problems: a practical guide for parents and teachers. London: David Fulton; 1997.

Novak, Julie C. (1999). Novak: Ingalls & Salerno's Maternal & Child Health Nursing, 9th ed., St. Louis, MO: Mosby.

Opperman, C. & Cassandra, K. (1998). Contemporary Pediatric Nursing, St. Louis, MO: Mosby.

Orr D. Helping adolescents toward adulthood. Contemp Pediatr 1998; 15(5): 55-76.

Pamela A. (1999). Nursing Care of Infants and Children, 6th ed., St. Louis, MO: Mosby.

Pilliterri, Adele. (2003). Maternal and Child Health Nursing, 4th ed., Philadelphia, PA: J. B. Lippincott.

Prazar G, Friedman S. An office-based approach to adolescent psychosocial issues. Contemp Pediatr 1997; 14(5):59-76.

Rudolph MC, Levene MI. Paediatrics and child health. Oxford: Blackwell Science; 1999.

Rudy C. Developmental dysplasia of the hip: what's new in the 1990's. J Pediatr Health Care 1996; 10(2):85.

Schulte, Elizabeth B., Price, Debra L., & Gwin, Julie F. (2001). Thompson's Pediatric Nursing, 8th ed., Philadelphia, PA: W. B. Saunders.

Taylor J, Muller D. Nursing adolescents: research and psychological perspectives. Oxford: Blackwell Sciences; 1995.

Thomas DO. Assessing children-it's different. RN 1996; 59(4):38-44.

Vessey JA. Developmental approaches to examining young children. Pediatr Nurs 1995;21(l):53-56.

Viner R. Youth matters. London: Action for Sick Children; 1999.

White, Lois. (2002) Basic Nursing Foundations of Skills and Concepts, Albany, NY: Delmar Publishing.

Wong D. Nursing care of infants and children, 6th edn. St. Louis: Mosby; 1999.

Wong DL, Wilson D. Whaley and Wong's nursing care of infants and children, 6th edn. St. Louis: Mosby; 1999.

Wong DL. The paper doll technique. Pediatr Nurs 1981; 7:39-40.

Wong, Donna L. (1997). Whaley & Wong's Essentials of Pediatric Nursing, 5th ed., St. Louis, MO: Mosby.

# Index